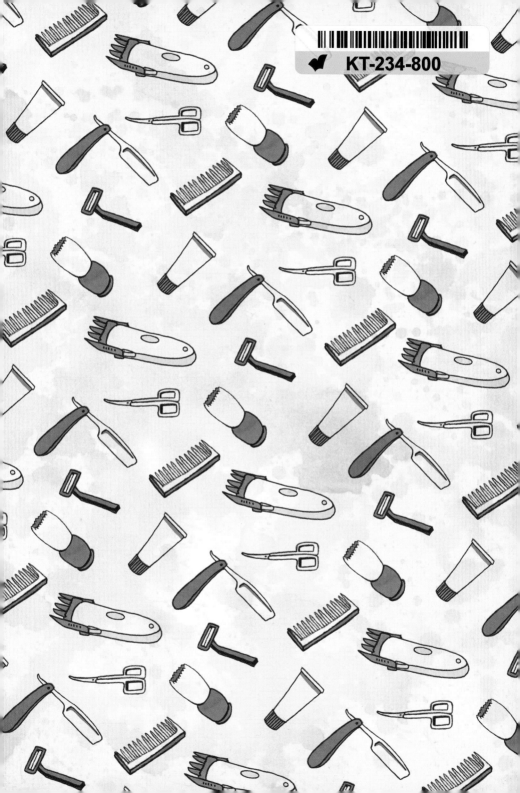

THIS BEARDED LIFE

CARLES SUÑÉ   ALFONSO CASAS

Quarto is the authority on a wide range of topics.
Quarto educates, entertains and enriches the lives of
our readers – enthusiasts and lovers of hands-on living.
www.QuartoKnows.com

First published in the UK in 2016 by
Aurum Press Limited
74-77 White Lion Street
London N1 9PF
www.QuartoKnows.com

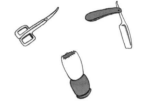

First published in Spanish in 2015 by Lunwerg
Editorial Planeta, S.A.
Avenida Diagonal, 662-662 – 08034
Barcelona
Spain

Copyright © 2016 Alfonso Casas and Carles Suñé
Text by Carles Suñé
www.nosinmibarba.com
Translation by Elena Feehan
Illustrations by Alfonso Casas
www.alfonsocasas.tumblr.com
Design and layout by temabcn
www.temabcn.com

A catalogue record for this book is available from the British Library.

ISBN 978 1 78131 601 6

10 9 8 7 6 5 4 3 2 1
2020 2019 2018 2017 2016

Printed in China

THIS BEARDED LIFE

CARLES SUÑÉ ALFONSO CASAS

Aurum
Press

CONTENTS

MEN'S *LIFESTYLE* – WITH A HAIRY DIFFERENCE

If I had to pinpoint the moment when my passion for beards began, I would say it was when I got promoted to a senior position at the company I used to work for. All my colleagues were older than me and I needed to give off a certain air of authority. A beard was the obvious solution – but I soon realised that sporting facial hair not only gave me more presence; I also really liked how it looked. That was when I knew that my beard was to become an integral part of who I was.

Time has passed and it has remained ever thus. We've had moments where we've drifted a little, my beard and I, but our relationship can withstand anything. Indeed, by some strange twist of fate, the moment I got married – the moment I made a solemn commitment to my partner – coincided almost exactly with the moment I made a not dissimilar commitment to my beard: I decided to start a blog called *No sin mi barba* – literally, 'Not without my beard' in English.

What began as a way to cope with a radical change in lifestyle when I moved from Barcelona to A Coruña, quickly turned into a men's lifestyle website – but with beards as a leitmotiv. The site got such a fantastic reception right from the off that I realised it had been launched at just the right time; that this was the beard's time to shine.

As the project went from strength to strength, I received a call from Lunwerg offering me the chance to collaborate with Alfonso Casas on a new project: a book. How could I refuse?

This Bearded Life is not so much a guide as a style handbook. Chapter by chapter, we'll be exploring a phenomenon which may, for some, be nothing more than a passing trend, but which, for us, is a whole lot more. For us, it is an attitude, a way of life – one we would like to share with you.

We're not claiming this to be any kind of great philosophical essay, or an in-depth dermatology lecture, or a hyper-intellectual scientific study on the subject of facial hair. All we want to do is take a look at how beards have been represented and perceived over the years: day-to-day matters, how the bearded man's image has evolved, how beards became a business opportunity,

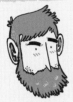

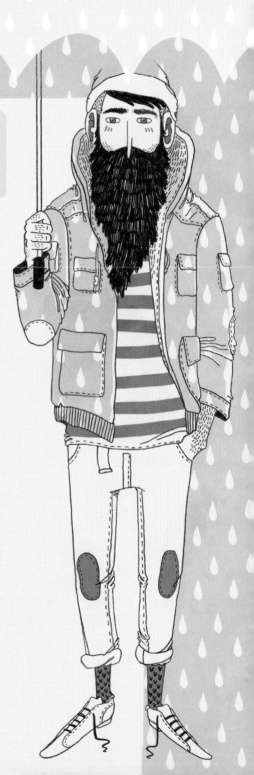

and a guide to who's who in the world of facial hair.

This book reflects the new way of life for the beared man. A way of life we love, which revolves around the principles I've shared on my website, and one that has no qualms about shouting from the rooftops that 'a beard is more than just facial hair; it's an attitude, a cornerstone of masculinity'. And the time has come to explain what that way of life is all about.

This Bearded Life is an interesting collection of observations, musings, advice and recommendations about the world of beards, barbers, and the bearded masses. Its structure, its informative content and its photos and illustrations make this book something akin to a style guide, a how-to manual and a collector's item all rolled into one – perfect for beard connoisseurs, for experts and for the curious, and for those with a simply undeniable affinity for all things facial hair.

We've loved every moment of making this book a reality, and we hope that you enjoy it every bit as much.

Here's to this bearded life!

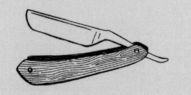

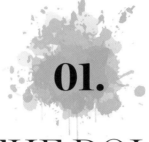

01.

THE ROLE
OF BEARDS
IN CULTURE
AND SOCIETY

---

*The relationship between men and beards
dates back to the very beginning
of our existence*

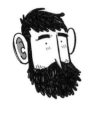

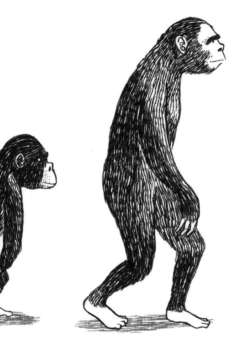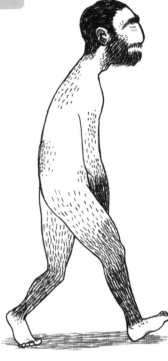

'TO GIVE UP ONE'S BEARD IS TO GIVE UP MAN'S MOST FUNDAMENTAL ESSENCE: HIS HAIR.'

The relationship between men and beards dates back to the very beginning of our existence. Our faces and other body parts were already covered in hair long before we even learned to walk upright. Throughout their meandering history, beards have taken up residence on the faces of countless men, from pharaohs, to Greek philosophers, to absolutist monarchs. Some even claim that, in early forms of civilisation, only shamans were entrusted with the responsibility of looking after the beards and hair of their cave-dwelling fellow citizens.

Indeed, the role of barber was once such a position of responsibility that, during the Middle Ages, in addition to trimming beards and cutting hair, barbers also carried out tasks usually associated with other professions: taking out teeth, treating patients with cataracts and hernias, drawing blood, and even removing tumours. Fortunately, these practices became much better regulated once the 15th century began, and eventually they were taken out of barbers' hands altogether.

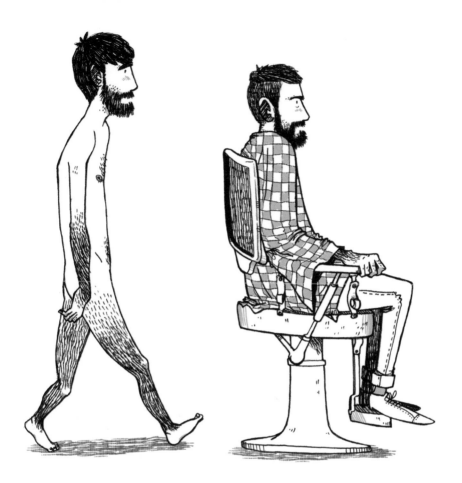

Under the influence of the Roman and Carolingian Empires, beards were demonized for many centuries. Anyone seen sporting one was considered, at best, a slob or, at worst, an atheist, and some were even excommunicated. Luckily, the passage of time softened this radical approach, and during periods such as the Renaissance and the Victorian era, beards once again became a sign of sophistication and elegance.

But if there has been any point at which beards have truly taken centre stage, it's the 20th century – and now the 21st as well. In the 1940s and '50s, bikers began using beards as a demonstration of identity; and the '60s saw the birth of the hippie movement, among whose members beards took on an almost mystical quality. Today, beards are making a Madonna-esque comeback thanks to the rise of hipsters, lumbersexuals and the Twitter generation. But what kind of future lies ahead for our beloved facial hair?

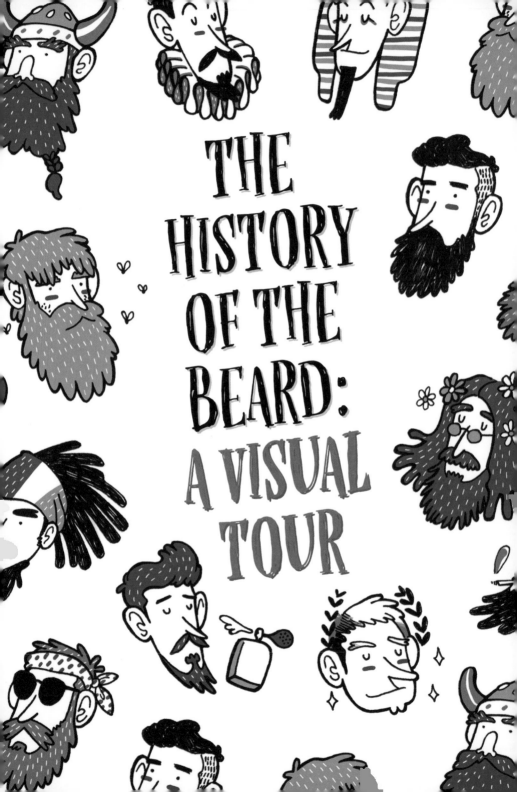

THE HISTORY OF THE BEARD:

A VISUAL TOUR

MESOPOTAMIA, EGYPT, GREECE AND THE VIKINGS

For the Akkadians and the Assyrians, beards were a symbol of authority. The same was true of the Egyptians, whose pharaohs used to braid gold threads into their facial hair. For the Greeks, beards represented wisdom, and in Viking culture they were sacred: any Viking who trimmed his beard was sent into exile. They would sign agreements in which they swore never to cut their facial hair, and in many cases their beards earned them nicknames.

Popularity level: 🧔 🧔 🧔 🧔

ROMANS AND CAROLINGIANS

The Romans stamped out beards, believing them to indicate slovenliness and a lack of hygiene. As the Church gradually gained more and more power, it pushed for beards to be deemed a sign of paganism. This contempt for facial hair reached its zenith under the Carolingian Empire, when Pope Gregory VII issued an edict declaring that 'bearded men would be excommunicated from the Church'.

Popularity level: 0

THE RENAISSANCE AND THE VICTORIAN ERA

The Renaissance saw facial hair begin to make a comeback. Members of the French court sported short, carefully maintained beards styled using wax – a fashion which was quickly taken up by the masses. It was the Victorian era, however, which truly experienced a facial hair boom: moustaches, mutton chops and long, pointed beards were deemed the very height of refinement and sophistication.

Popularity level: 🧔 🧔 🧔

HIPPIES, RASTAFARIANS AND BIKERS

Cultural movements and the rise of urban tribes transformed beards into a demonstration of identity. For hippies, it was a sign of freedom, for Rastafarians a show of adherence to Old Testament law, and for bikers it was a symbol of identity and community.

Popularity level: 🧔 🧔 🧔 🧔

21ST CENTURY: HIPSTERS AND OTHER TRENDY TYPES

Although the beard's current fashionable status is thought to have started with hipsters – a social subculture whose primary haunts include New York's Soho and Brooklyn, as well as London's Shoreditch – they're certainly not the only ones getting a piece of the action. Hipsters' appropriation of facial hair has made beards more mainstream and, as a result, has given the traditional barber's profession a new lease of life, as well as creating a market for associated products and services.

Popularity level: 🧔 🧔 🧔 🧔 🧔 🧔 🧔 🧔 🧔

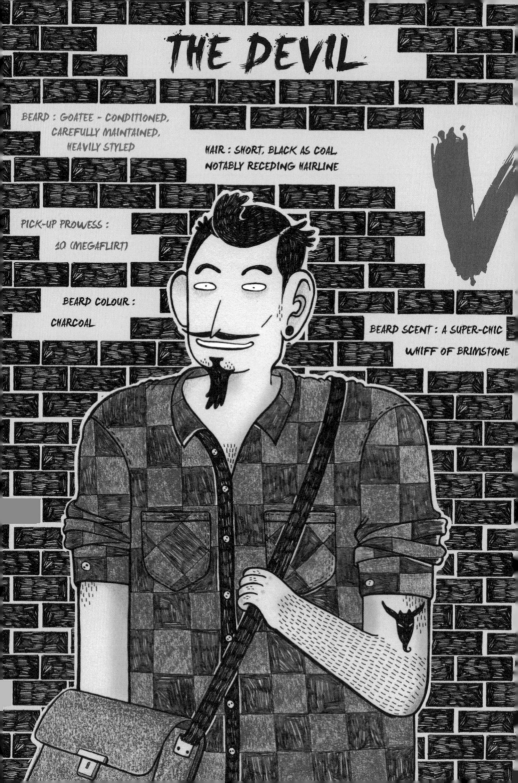

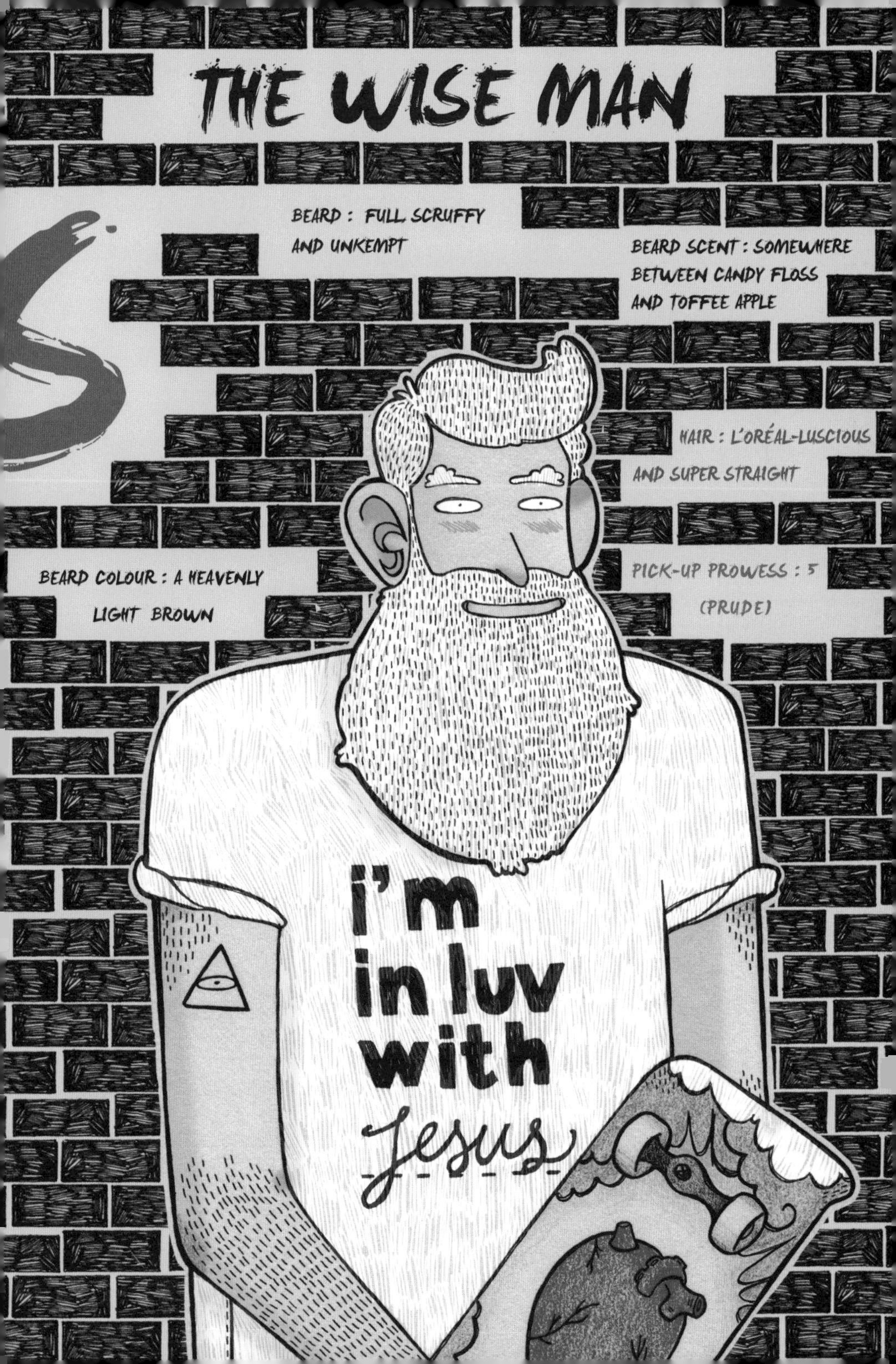

THE WISE MAN

BEARD : FULL SCRUFFY
AND UNKEMPT

BEARD SCENT : SOMEWHERE
BETWEEN CANDY FLOSS
AND TOFFEE APPLE

HAIR : L'ORÉAL-LUSCIOUS
AND SUPER STRAIGHT

BEARD COLOUR : A HEAVENLY
LIGHT BROWN

PICK-UP PROWESS : 5
(PRUDE)

i'm
in luv
with
Jesus

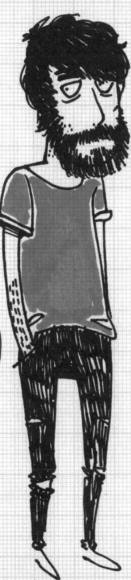

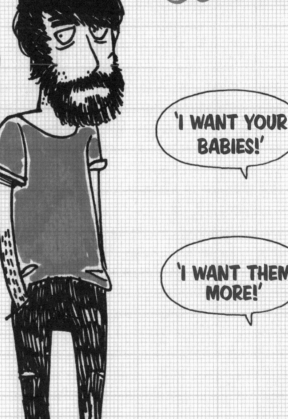

MODERN BEARDS
AND SOCIAL MOVEMENTS

*From the hippies of San Francisco to the hipsters of Sant Antoni –
via a few biker gangs...*

The 20th century's various social movements proved a fertile breeding ground for a number of different subcultures. Though what united the members of these urban tribes were shared ideologies and interests, they also shared a common aesthetic of which beards were a key part – which led to facial hair becoming a sign of union, of belonging to a group.

Let's take a look back at the latter years of the 1940s, when motorcycle aficionados began to gather in huge groups whose main characteristics were leather, beards and big-ass bikes. Indeed, it is commonly believed that 1948 saw the birth in Los Angeles of the largest and most famous biker gang, Hell's Angels, for whom beards were more important than the engines of their powerful two-wheeled toys.

If we then skip ahead to the end of the '60s, we arrive at the moment which epitomised the hippie movement: Woodstock, 1969 – a festival held in Bethel, New York, despite the fact that the roots of the movement lay (and lie still) in San Francisco. Hippie beards,

for their part, were borne of a combination of laziness, a desire for whimsy over military neatness, and a penchant for all things natural.

Fast-forwarding now to the present day, the trendiest parts of some of the world's major capital cities – Shoreditch on one side of the Atlantic; Williamsburg on the other – have borne witness over the past four years to the emergence of the hipster, wearing his beard like a badge of honour. As time has passed, new breeds of hipster have developed, their profile slightly different to that of the original and their style choices dictated more by fashion than anything else. Take twees, for example: sporting a fresh-faced take on the hipster look, twees love the films of directors like Wes Anderson and Spike Jonze and tend to be hyper eco-conscious. Lumbersexuals, meanwhile, are similarly green-minded, but their look is more manly-woodcutter-meets-stylish-hipster. Not forgetting, of course, the part-hippie-part-hipster 'trend' (cold fusion, more like) of adorning one's beard with flowers...

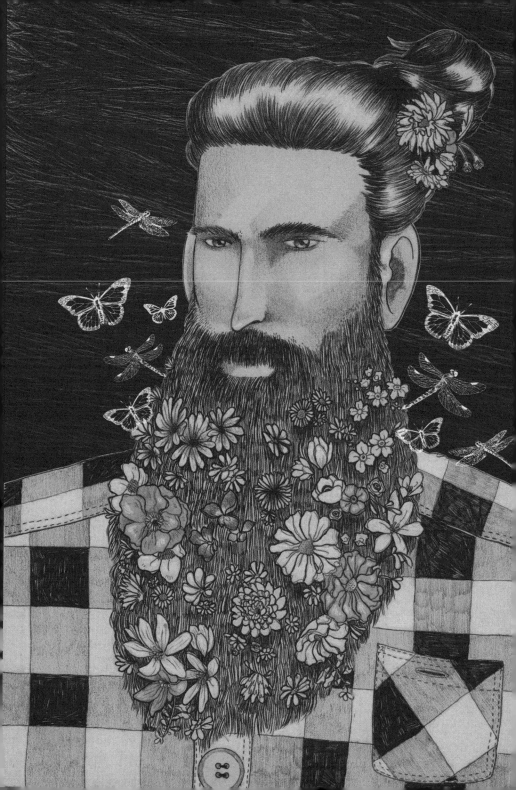

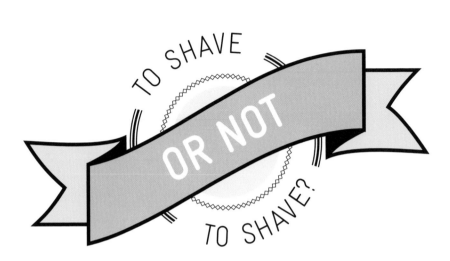

TO SHAVE

OR NOT

TO SHAVE?

The diktats of fashion are as rigid as they are bizarre. Everyone wants to be *à la mode* – to be the it-girl or it-boy who's bang on trend – and when it comes to facial hair, we're no different. They're ubiquitous right now – but for how long? Are beards just a fashion statement, or are they part of our identity?

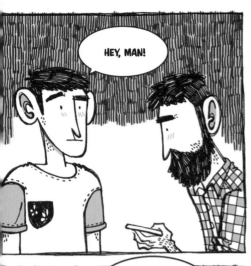

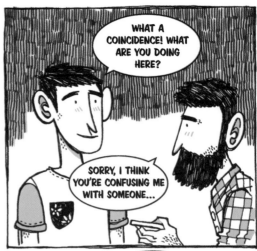

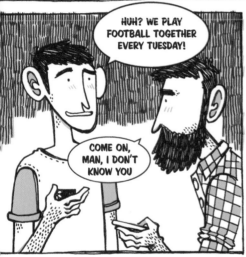

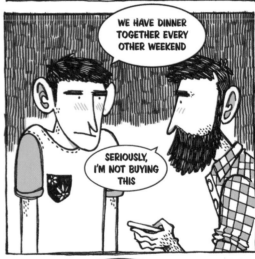

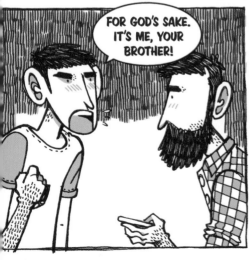

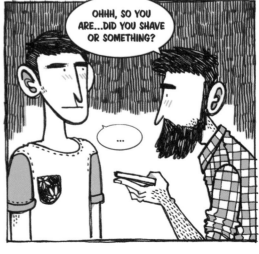

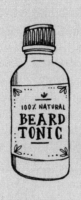

02.

THE CURRENT BEARDED CLIMATE

*The past five years have seen
the start of a golden age for beards*

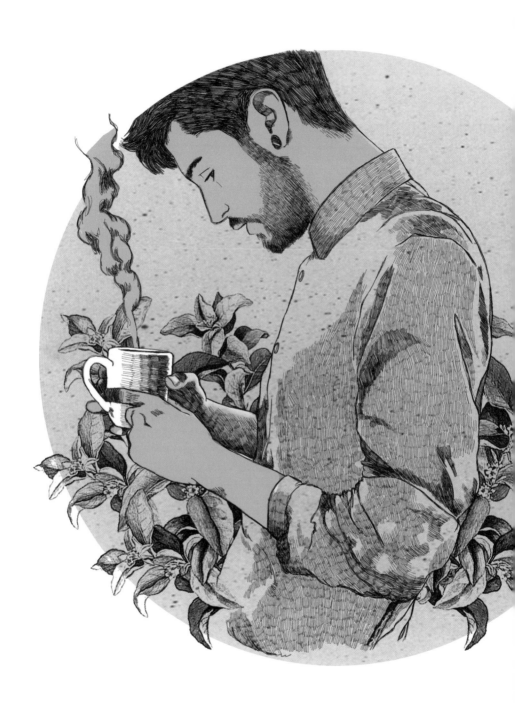

The past five years have seen the start of a veritable golden age for beards. The rise of facial hair in the majority of Western countries, Spain in particular, is indisputable – a boom rivalled only by the ones experienced by that most genteel and traditional of beverages, the gin and tonic, and by that most deliciously fattening and deliriously sugary of treats, the cupcake.

The reasons why men decide to grow their beards are as numerous as the individuals who have done so in recent years: because they want one, plain and simple; to hide facial flaws; to try and be different (or so they think); or merely to follow what they believe to be nothing more than a passing trend. Whatever each individual's motivation, the reality is that men are becoming more and more image-conscious – giving rise to a number of new male style archetypes, which we're going to examine in this chapter. We'll start with metrosexuality – the trend which declared war on male body hair: leg hair, pubic hair, facial hair – even eyebrows. We'll also be taking a look at 'ubersexuals', who have reclaimed the *au naturel* look, with their three-day beards and deceptively high-maintenance haircuts; 'lumbersexuals', the ultimate embodiment of rugged rural style; and what we've dubbed 'barbosexuals' – men whose beards (or *barbas*, in Spanish, hence the nickname) are their BFFs. Beards are now so present in our everyday lives that there's no getting away from them. They're all over Instagram – rivalling photos of kittens, food, and feet on the beach – and the worlds of both cinema and advertising are falling over themselves to capitalise on their appeal. In short, dear readers, we are living in the age of the beard.

As of about four years ago, it's now nigh on impossible to find a bar whose menu doesn't list a wide range of unique takes on the traditional gin and tonic. The same is true of cupcakes: anywhere that's anywhere now offers these sweet treats in every shape, colour and flavour under the sun. Now it's beards that are taking centre stage, and there are plenty of men that are keen to get in on the action.

THE RISE OF THE G&T...

It's official: the gin and tonic is the drink of the moment – preferably served with half a salad in the glass. And if you don't know which tonic works best with which gin or which are the top brands – well, better start doing your homework.

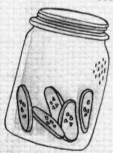
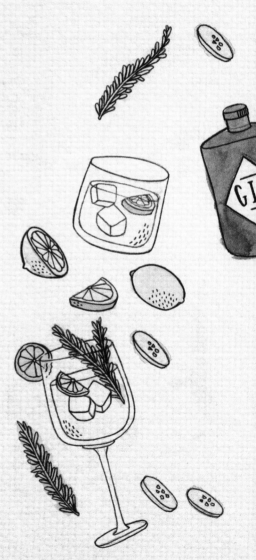
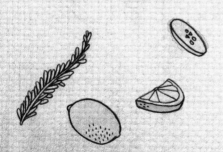

...THE CUPCAKE...

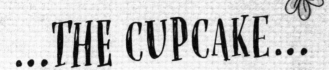

The trendy areas of any city worth its salt are now teeming with top-heavy fairy cakes covered with enormous dollops of icing – otherwise known as cupcakes. But beware: they may be small, but they don't half pack a punch in the sugar stakes.

...AND THE BEARD?

Until as recently as just five years ago, beards were a relatively rare sight, and if you did happen to pass a man with a lot of facial hair, you'd turn

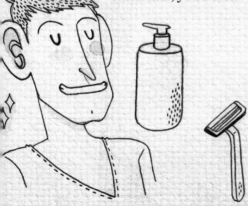

to get a closer look. Nowadays, though, they're ten a penny. It's fashionable to grow a big, bushy beard – and if it's paired with long hair pulled back in a 'man bun', so much the better.

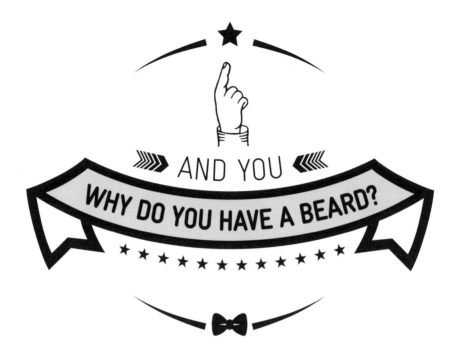

AND YOU
WHY DO YOU HAVE A BEARD?

Growing a beard is essentially a matter of time – and, admittedly, good genes, because let's face it, if your facial hair just doesn't grow, there's not much you can do about it besides hope for a miracle. So if you want to grow a thick, bushy beard, you have to devote a fair bit of time to it – at least three months, and at most...as long as you want! Getting rid of it is far easier after all: a quick shave and you're done.

The reasons why men decide to grow a beard are many and varied, but these are the top three: because they actively want one; because it's fashionable; or because they're lazy. While men in the first category have had beards pretty much from the moment they were born and would never dream of shaving them off, those in the second know that it's just a trend, and when beards are no longer fashionable they'll be reaching for the razor. The third kind of man is the most pragmatic: if he's got a beard, it's only because the mere thought of shaving fills him with lethargy. But it wouldn't be fair to only mention these three reasons for growing a beard, so let's take a look at a few more...

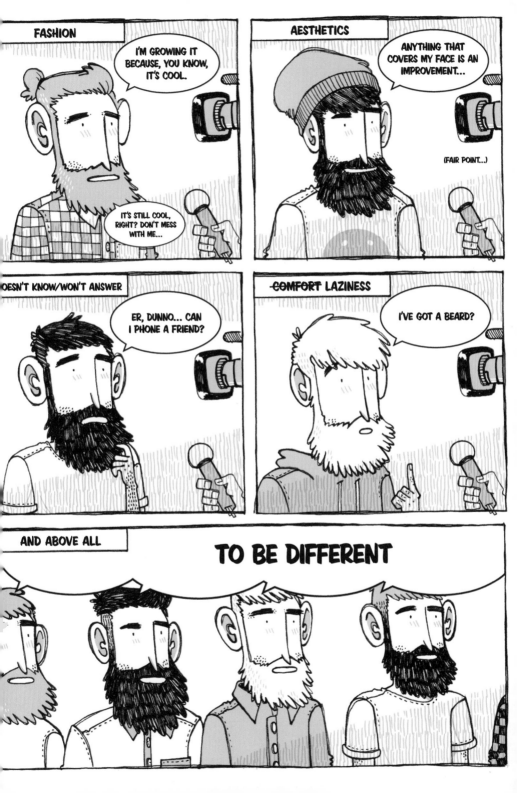

BEARDS AND TATTOOS

A potent combination?

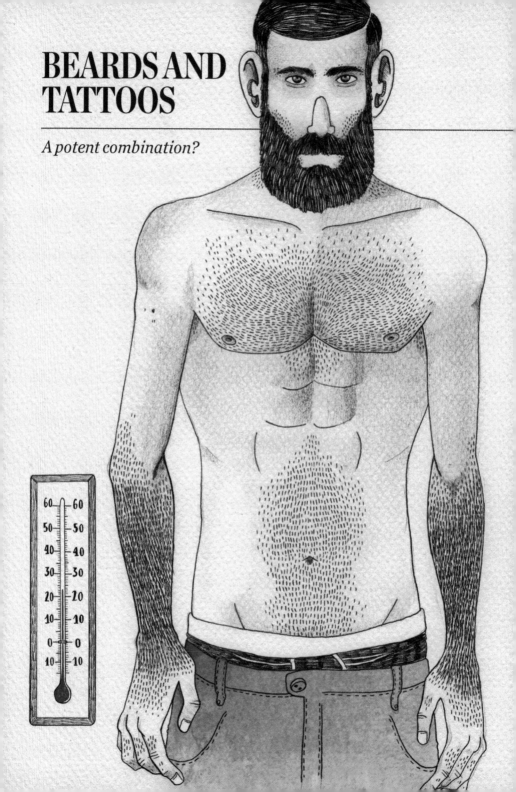

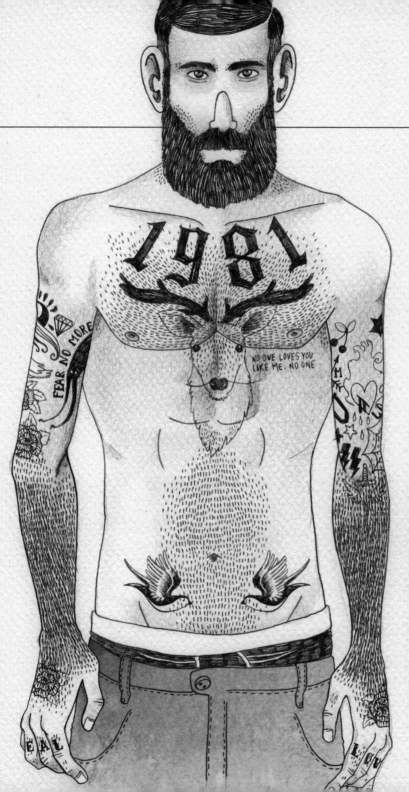
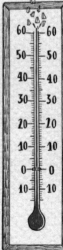

In our increasingly globalised world, new styles and social trends spread from country to country in the blink of an eye. Just look at how quickly the hipster trend took off around the globe, for instance. This context of globalisation has also allowed for a standardised series of male archetypes to emerge, with various celebrity examples serving as points of reference. If David Beckham was the metrosexual alpha male (nowadays it could also be Cristiano Ronaldo), George Clooney was and remains the standard-bearer for ubersexuality. Chuck Norris (more or less) fits the bill for an example of a famous lumbersexual, and in terms of an archetypal 'barbosexual' (a word we came up with ourselves), Ricky Hall, Billy Huxley and Christian Göran all spring readily to mind. Let's take a closer look at the main characteristics of each category:

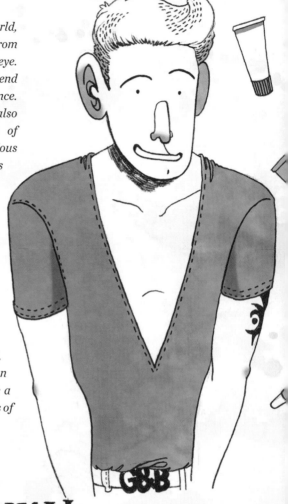

METROSEXUAL

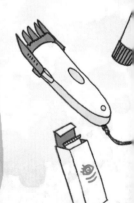

- ULTRA-PLUCKED EYEBROWS
- BLINGY PIERCINGS
- IMMACULATELY CLEAN-SHAVEN
- PLUNGING DEEP V-NECK
- BELT WITH OSTENTATIOUSLY LARGE BUCKLE

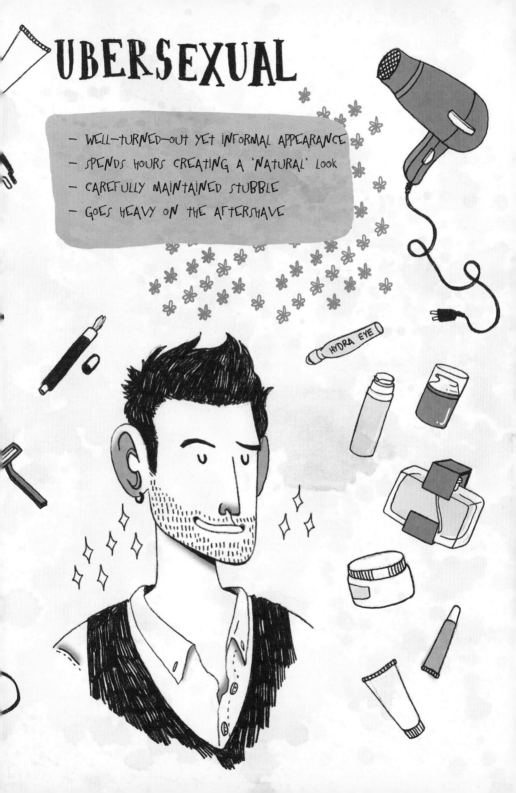

UBERSEXUAL

- WELL-TURNED-OUT YET INFORMAL APPEARANCE
- SPENDS HOURS CREATING A 'NATURAL' LOOK
- CAREFULLY MAINTAINED STUBBLE
- GOES HEAVY ON THE AFTERSHAVE

HYDRA EYE

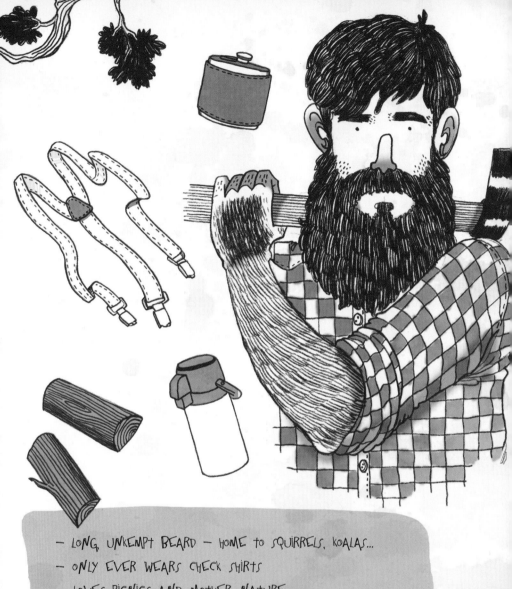

- LONG, UNKEMPT BEARD — HOME TO SQUIRRELS, KOALAS...
- ONLY EVER WEARS CHECK SHIRTS
- LOVES PICNICS AND MOTHER NATURE
- LIVES INSIDE A REDWOOD TREE

LUMBER SEXUAL

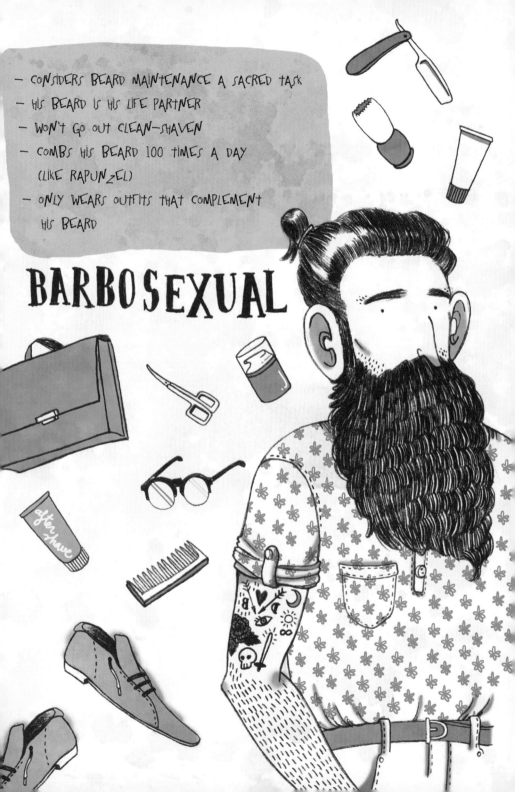

- CONSIDERS BEARD MAINTENANCE A SACRED TASK
- HIS BEARD IS HIS LIFE PARTNER
- WON'T GO OUT CLEAN-SHAVEN
- COMBS HIS BEARD 100 TIMES A DAY
  (LIKE RAPUNZEL)
- ONLY WEARS OUTFITS THAT COMPLEMENT
  HIS BEARD

BARBOSEXUAL

INSTAGRAM

A world of kittens, foodies, feet and beards

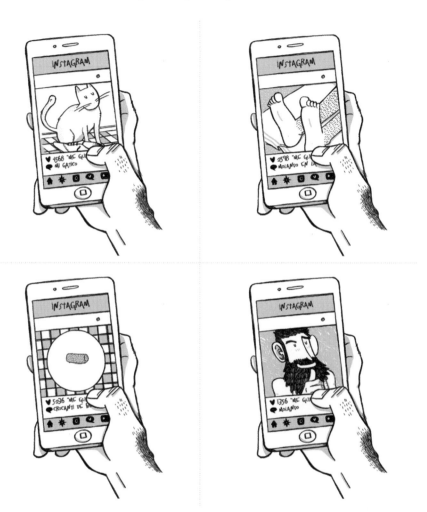

Instagram has made cats an inescapable part of our everyday lives, thanks to the countless kitty photos uploaded to the network every day. It's also the playground of thousands of foodies, plus the usual suspects looking to make the world jealous with photos of their feet enjoying some Caribbean beach or other. But if there's anyone that's really taking Instagram by storm – getting Likes by the thousand – it's guys with beards (hot guys, mainly, of course).

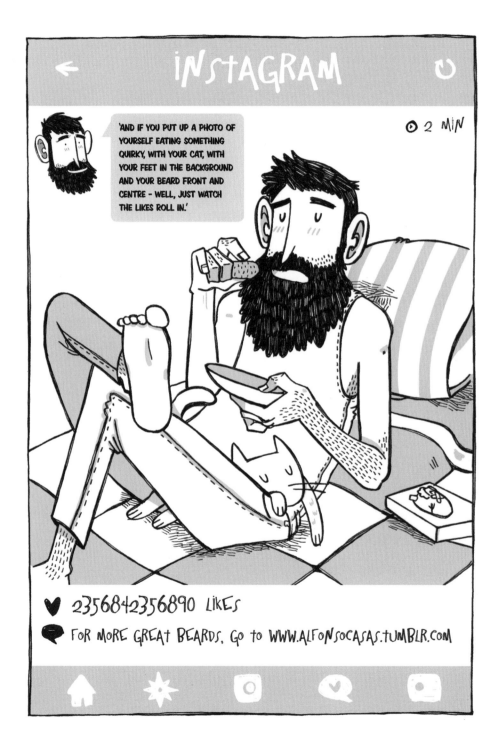

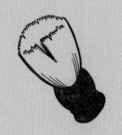

03.

BEARD
BUSINESS

---

*Any new trend brings with it
new business opportunities*

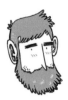

Generally speaking, any new fashion or trend brings with it new business opportunities. If the G&T has brought back cocktail bars, and cupcakes have brought about the flourishing success of hundreds of Instagrammable cafés and brunch spots, the beard boom has given traditional barbers a chance to rediscover their former glory. The classic neighbourhood barber's is back in the limelight, offering brand new services and dusting off old-fashioned ones like the classic shave. In just a short period of time, the industry has transformed itself: closing ranks, becoming stronger and more unified, with barbers dubbing themselves lofty titles and organising conferences, courses and events right, left and centre – and all with beards as their primary focus.

Alongside the rise of the barber, a new market for special beard and moustache maintenance products has emerged and is growing at an extraordinary rate. These products are now well established in Scandinavia and the English-speaking world, but Spain is still relying largely on imports to supply the growing demand from shops and websites jumping on the beard bandwagon. In terms of home-grown Spanish manufacturing, we've arrived very late to the party, with so far just a couple of brands producing anything for the beard market.

Nevertheless, neither of these new business opportunities would exist had the general public not taken to the new beard trend so readily – even though initially it seemed to be the preserve only of a select subculture. This process of acceptance and mainstreaming has required some people to overcome long-standing facial hair prejudices: to go from rejecting beards on the basis that they make you look older, to understanding that they can actually make you more attractive. After that, it wasn't long before the world discovered that bearded men tend to have a better sex life (a matter we'll be looking at more closely in the next chapter), and before we knew it, we had accepted them not only as a vital feature of the male facial landscape, but as something to love and care for too.

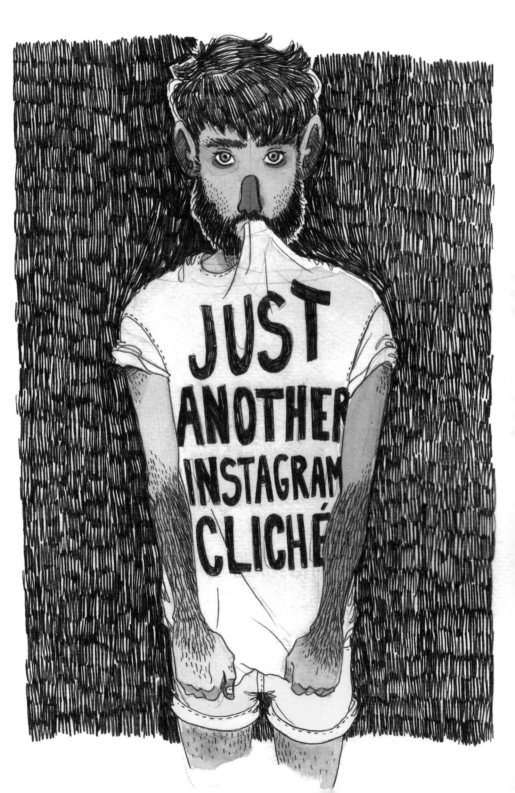

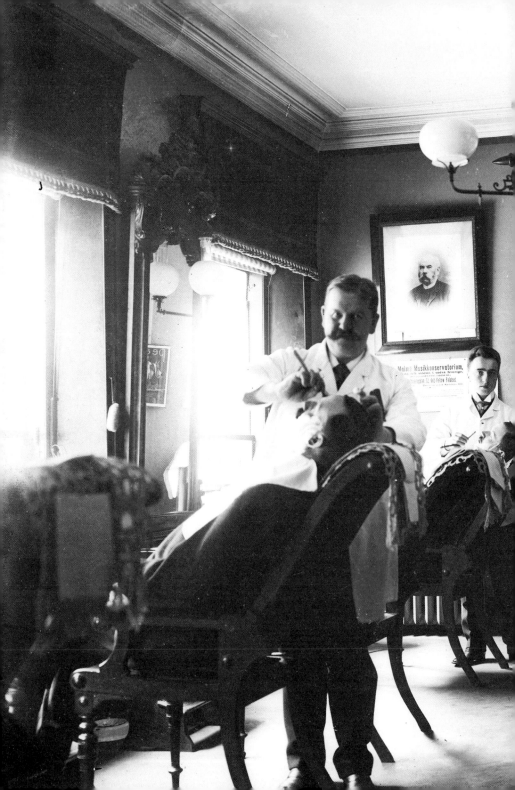

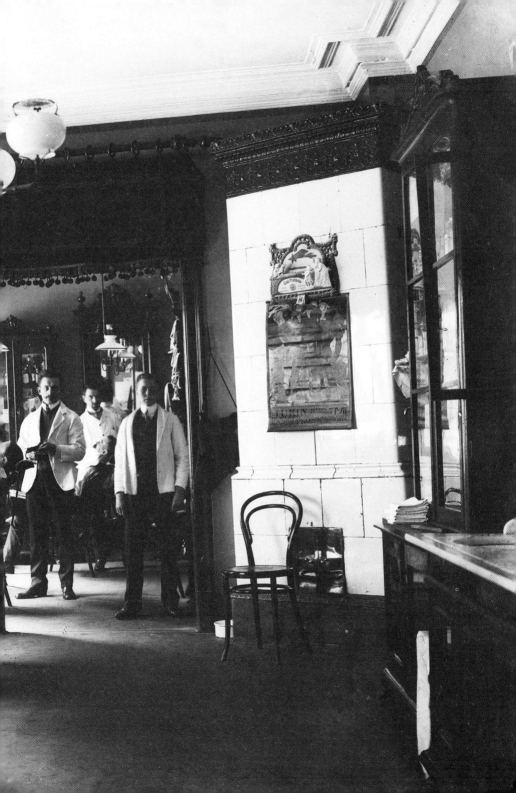

THE BARBERSHOP REVIVAL

The emergence of fashions and trends always brings about a certain amount of economic activity. Sometimes entirely new markets are created – like the e-cigarette market currently on the rise. In other cases, however, pre-existing industries are simply taken down off the shelf and given a new lease of life – which is precisely what has happened to the traditional barbershop. Though barbers already have a long and rich history, they have recently undergone a full 21st century transformation, and now more and more people are looking to open a barber's of their own. All this in just a few short years.

2010

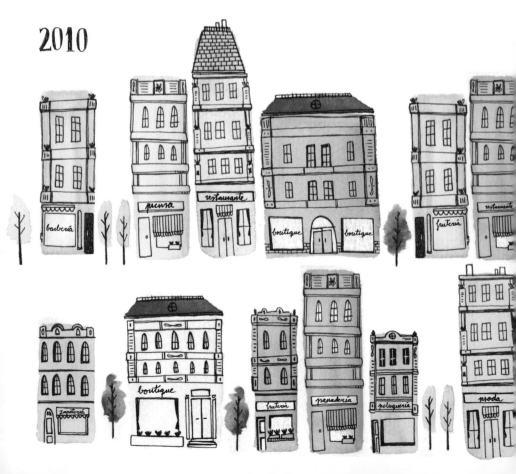

Yet getting a few tattoos, acting edgy and opening a barber's that offers all the traditional services but with a cool, modern twist does not a real barber with a life's worth of experience make. Many people are taking advantage of the current craze to open up this kind of business, claiming skills and experience they simply don't possess. The same is true of training too. Nowadays, it seems anyone that wants to train budding barbers can do so, no matter whether or not they are genuinely qualified to educate others. It's become a vicious circle that's mostly an exercise in ego-stroking and in maintaining the status quo in an industry that's currently booming like never before.

And with barbers on the rise, so, too, are their prices: what would once have cost you four quid could now easily cost you forty. It's a question of supply and demand – and fashion, of course.

2015

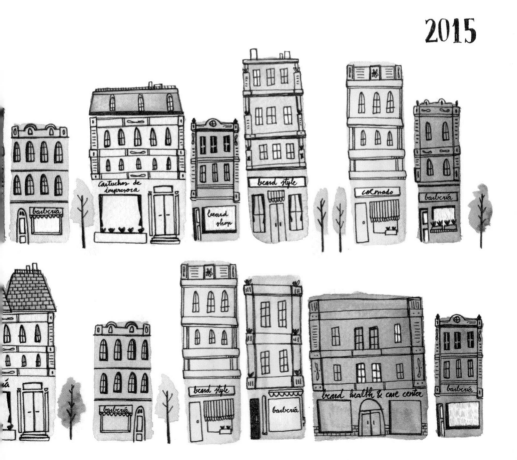

BEARD (AND MOUSTACHE) CARE PRODUCTS

Another business opportunity provided by the beard boom is the new market for products specifically designed for facial hair.

Modern men are taking increasing care over their appearance, especially those of us with beards we'd like to keep looking tidy, healthy and smelling heavenly. Luckily, there are now a number of products available to help us do just that.

BEARD SOAP

Contrary to what people may believe, the hair in your beard is not the same as the hair on your head. It's much coarser, and it tends to make the skin it grows out of become dry. Beards also get dirty easily, with a tendency to pick up not just bad smells (cigarette smoke, etc.) but also bits of food. For this reason, it's important to wash and hydrate your beard daily – for the good of both your hair and your skin.

BEARD BALM

It is precisely because beards can cause dry skin that we need to keep them well hydrated. Products such as beard balms – especially ones with a high percentage of natural ingredients – are excellent for conditioning and moisturizing facial hair to avoid skin becoming dry and flaky, and to prevent any hair loss or split ends in the beard itself. They come in plenty of scents, too.

BEARD OIL

Like beard balm, beard oil ensures that facial hair stays hydrated, as well as giving it a pleasant aroma. Some offer particular benefits – such as encouraging hair growth – or are specifically designed for certain hair types, and all provide a nice glossy finish.

WAX

Let's be honest – a good beard just isn't the same without a good moustache to go with it, so it's important to look after them both. Special moustache waxes (though some choose to use them on their beards, too) allow you to shape your 'tache into whatever style you fancy, be it something classic or something a little more Dalí-esque.

BRUSHES

There are all kinds of brushes on offer – ones for different beard lengths, ones especially for moustaches, and so on – but all of them are excellent tools for giving facial hair shape and body.

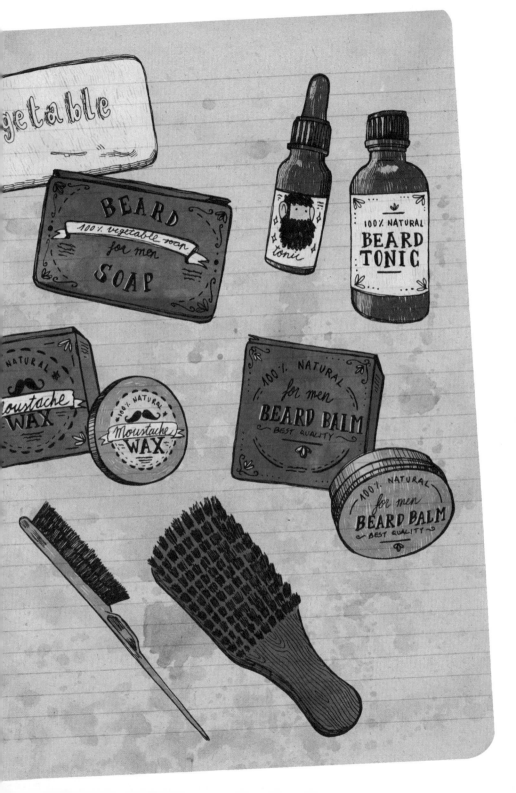

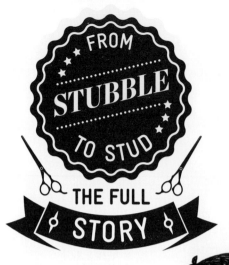

FROM STUBBLE ~~STUBBLE~~ TO STUD

THE FULL STORY

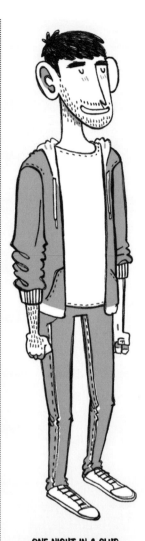

TEENAGERS DO IT ~~BETTER~~ DO IT DO IT & DO IT

YOU STARTED SHAVING DAILY BECAUSE HAVING A BEARD MAKES YOU LOOK OLDER AND YOU WANT TO STAY YOUNG FOREVER. EVEN THOUGH YOU'RE PUSHING 30, YOU STILL GET ASKED FOR ID WHEN YOU GO TO A BAR, YOU HAVE TO TAKE AN ADULT WITH YOU WHEN YOU WANT TO GET MONEY OUT AT THE BANK, AND YOU STILL HAVE TO ASK YOUR PARENTS' PERMISSION TO GO OUT PARTYING.

ONE NIGHT IN A CLUB, SOMEONE TELLS YOU THAT YOUR STUBBLE REALLY SUITS YOU AND MAKES YOU LOOK SEXY - SO YOU DECIDE TO KEEP IT. YOUR MUM, YOUR GRANDMA AND YOUR MORE AFFECTIONATE AUNTS TELL YOU THAT YOUR FACE IS SCRATCHY WHEN THEY KISS YOU, BUT YOU STAND YOUR GROUND: NO SHAVING.

SO YOU'VE GOT YOUR STUBBLE, BUT WHEREAS YOUR FULL-BEARDED FRIEND SEEMS TO BE HOOKING UP WITH SOMEONE EVERY WEEKEND, YOUR LUCK STILL HASN'T CHANGED. YOU WANT IN ON THE ACTION, SO YOU DECIDE TO GROW YOUR BEARD – AND IT WORKS! SOON YOU'RE A VERITABLE CASANOVA, AND YOUR INSTAGRAM LIKES ARE GOING THROUGH THE ROOF.

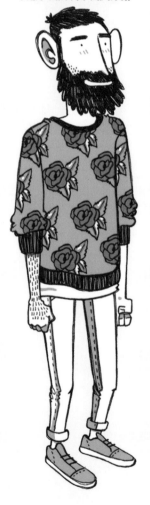

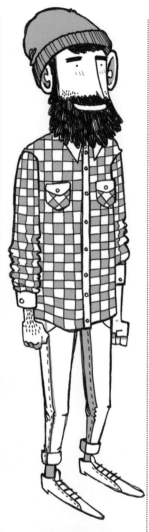

WITHIN THREE MONTHS, YOU'VE FILLED YOUR ENTIRE BATHROOM CABINET WITH BEARD PRODUCTS, YOU SEE YOUR BARBER MORE OFTEN THAN YOUR MOTHER, AND YOU'VE CHANGED YOUR RELATIONSHIP STATUS ON FACEBOOK TO 'ENGAGED TO MY BEARD'.

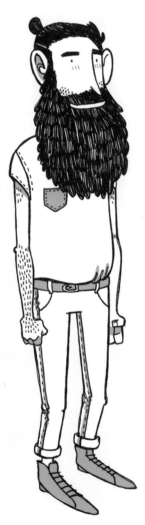

NOW THAT YOU'VE A WHOLE THICKET OF HAIR ON YOUR FACE, YOU REALISE THAT YOU NEED TO LOOK AFTER IT AND KEEP IT TIDY. SO YOU GO TO WWW. NOSINMIBARBA.COM, YOU READ EVERY SINGLE ARTICLE ON THERE ABOUT BEARD CARE, AND YOU BUY YOURSELF EVERY PRODUCT UNDER THE SUN.

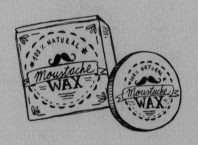

04.

THIS (DAILY) BEARDED LIFE

Having a beard is not as simple as just growing hair on your face and then forgetting about it

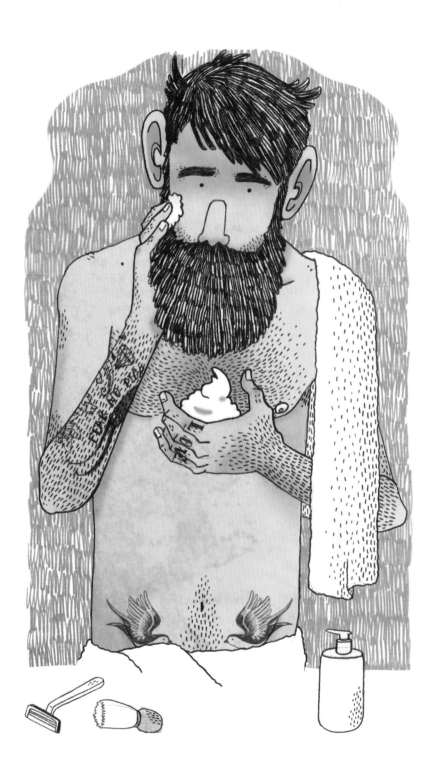

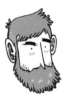

Having a beard is not as simple as just growing a load of hair all over your face and then forgetting about it. If you want a truly great beard, there are certain rituals that need to be carried out to encourage it to grow both longer and healthier. Both facial hair and the skin beneath it need washing daily, and also need to be kept hydrated. To help you do these things properly, there are (as we saw in the previous chapter) a number of products available specifically designed for beards, from special soaps and brushes, to waxes and oils. Over the next few pages, we're going to give you our top tips for keeping your beard – and moustache – clean and tidy, so that you always leave the house looking your best.

Now this might seem simple enough, but there are certain activities that are rather more difficult for the hairy of face. Eating, drinking, and even kissing all become much more complicated when you're trying not to get anything in your beard – or not to get your beard tangled in anything else.

In this chapter, we're also going to be taking a closer look at the classic fashion choices of our fellow bearded man: what they're wearing, what their wardrobe staples are, and which styles crop up again and again.

And, of course, we also want to talk about the day-to-day minutiae of this bearded life, and answer those questions so many of you have about whether bearded guys get more action, or whether we check each other out on the sly to see who's got the biggest beard...

A STEP-BY-STEP GUIDE TO BEARD (AND MOUSTACHE) CARE

When a guy decides to grow a beard – and we're talking a proper full beard here – he has two options: leave it to do its own thing and grow like a weed; or look after it so that it grows looking healthy, tidy and glossy. If you're going for the first option, you can skip this next section. If, however, it's the second option you're after, we're now going to explain how to care for your beautiful beard every day in just four simple steps.

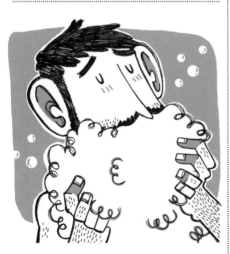

01.
WASHING

Washing your beard means adding an extra step to your daily shower routine, as well as an extra product: a special beard soap, the more natural ingredients the better. This is what you should use to wash both your beard and the skin beneath. It's just like washing the hair on your head: squeeze some soap onto your hands, then massage it carefully into your beard so that it forms a good lather for maximum effect. We recommend washing your beard towards the end of your shower, after you've washed your hair and body, as by this time the hot water will have opened up your pores, allowing the soap to work more effectively. Finish by rinsing thoroughly.

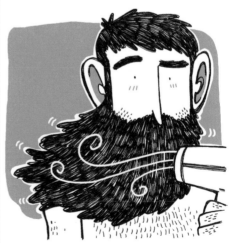

02.
DRYING

Once you're out of the shower, dry yourself, please, come on, else you'll freeze. Now remember, you can't just go towelling your beard dry like you would your hair – only use a towel to get rid of the excess moisture. Next, give it a blast of cold air with a hairdryer, but don't let it dry fully. Then, brush it gently and carefully to remove any knots or tangles.

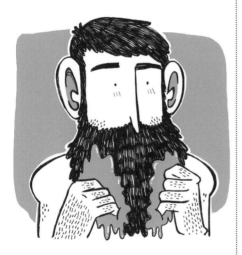

03.
HYDRATING

Now that your beard is nicely detangled with just a bit of moisture left, you can hydrate it with an oil or balm specially designed for beard care. If you're using an oil, put three or four drops onto your hands, rub them together, and then massage the oil into your beard. If you prefer balm, pop a small blob on your hands and apply as with oil. Bear in mind that the smell and shine that these oils and balms will give your beard will vary from product to product.

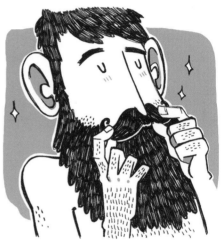

04.
SHAPING

Once you've applied your chosen conditioning product, you can comb your beard again, either with a brush or just with your fingers (don't overdo it though, or it can cause split ends). Now all that's left is the 'tache. Put a little wax on your fingertips, warm it up by rubbing your fingers gently together, and then apply it to your moustache, shaping it into your desired style. Now you're ready to go out and take on the world!

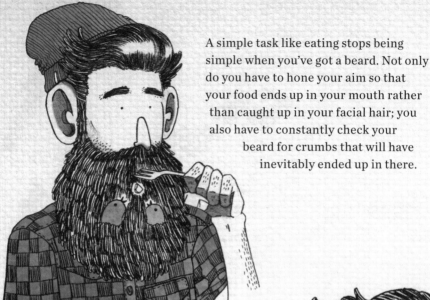

A simple task like eating stops being simple when you've got a beard. Not only do you have to hone your aim so that your food ends up in your mouth rather than caught up in your facial hair; you also have to constantly check your beard for crumbs that will have inevitably ended up in there.

EAT DRINK LOVE

Although having a beard can be awesome, it can sometimes make life complicated – rendering simple tasks trickier than a challenge on Takeshi's Castle. Here are just three examples of difficult situations with which we bearded folk have to contend.

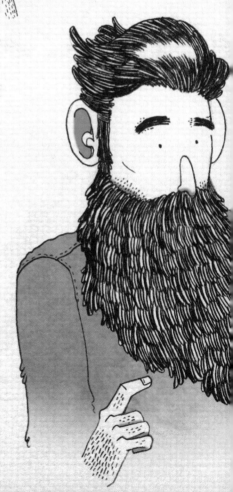

Drinking isn't that easy either. Enjoying a pint can be a complete headache when you're trying to avoid your moustache getting covered in foam. The solution is to always carry a straw with you, so that you can drink whatever you fancy without making a mess – though for coffee there are actually even special cups designed to protect moustaches, which have been around since the 18th century.

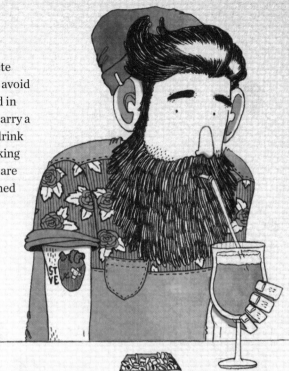

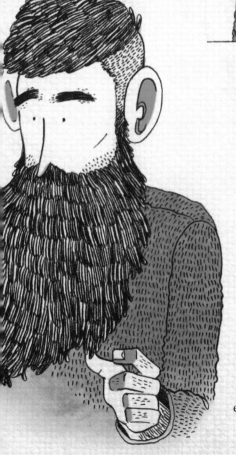

Beards even find a way to cause problems in...intimate situations. Though many people consider facial hair a feature which increases a guy's sex appeal, and in some circumstances it can cause a very enjoyable tickling sensation, in others it's more of a hindrance than a help. One of the most feared beard-related mood-killers – for men and women alike – is the so called 'Velcro effect' – need we say more?

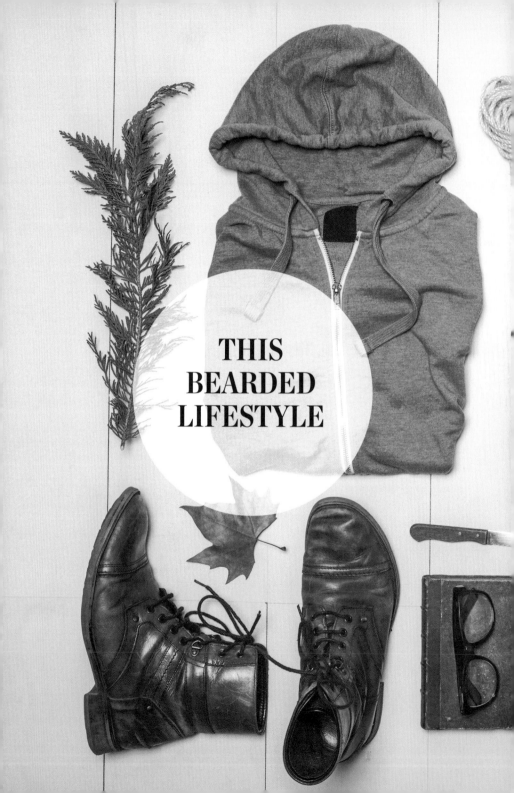

THIS
BEARDED
LIFESTYLE

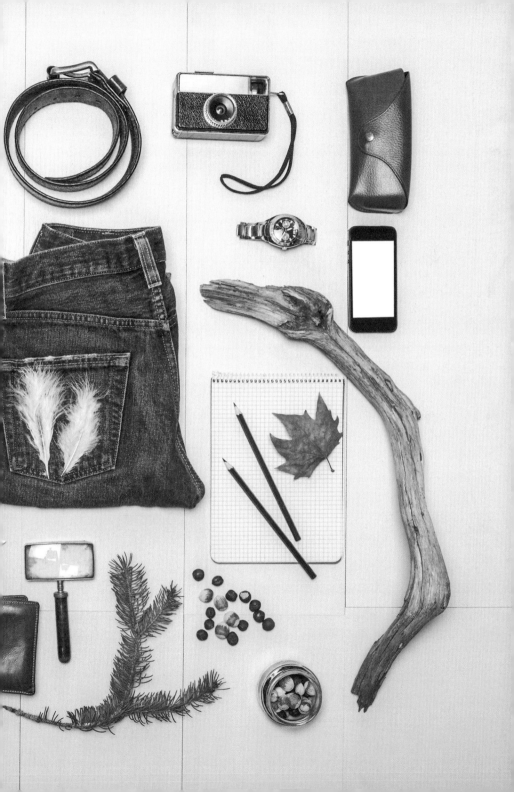

In chapter 2, we looked at the variety of reasons why guys decide to grow beards, as well as talking about 'barbosexuals' – so called because, well, we invented the word. For the barbosexual, having a beard is about more than just having hair on his face; it's a state of mind, one that manifests itself through many different aspects of his everyday life – particularly his clothes and accessories.

BEARDED BASICS

WOOLLY HAT

A wardrobe staple for any bearded hipster. If you want to dial the hipster vibe down a notch or two, a snapback (a baseball cap with a wide, flat peak) is also an option, or failing that – and if accompanied by a couple of other lumbersexual touches – long hair pulled back into a Samurai-style man bun.

CHECK SHIRT OR BRETON TEE

It'll depend on the overall style of the man in question as to which of these he opts for. If it's an outdoorsy look he likes, he'll be wearing the check shirt; if he's more into the nautical vibe, it'll be the striped Breton tee.

KNITTED JUMPER

Another fashion must, the knitted jumper is bang on trend and looks great

paired with a big, bushy beard. No barbosexual wardrobe is complete without one, preferably with a tribal or ethnic print.

PARKA, TRENCH OR FULL-LENGTH COAT

Of these three coat options, bearded blokes working a more modern look tend to plump for the parka – versatile and full of character. Those with more classic leanings are more likely to go for a trench coat or failsafe mac, or even a long coat with wide, flamboyant lapels.

JEGGINGS, CHINOS OR SKINNY JEANS

A bearded man's choice of legwear will, once again, depend on how modern his style is. Jeggings (a cross between jeans and leggings) are perfect for those who like to be able to move – skaters, for example, many of whom do tend to sport beards. Meanwhile, chinos or skinny jeans, preferably with the bottoms turned up a little, are the ideal option for a more classic look.

BACKPACK

Cross-body bags aren't cool anymore, men's handbags even less so. Nope, nowadays it's all about backpacks – preferably square ones, and either one block colour or in some kind of ethnic-look print. Those new to the bearded party will carry a backpack around empty but for their keys and wallet – but a veteran will always remember to pop some beard oil in his, to keep his beard hydrated throughout the day, and a brush to keep it looking shipshape.

SHOES OR TRAINERS

For the beard enthusiast who puts being chic above all else, it has to be the classic, Italian-style leather brogues, with toes that strike just the right balance between pointed and rounded. Those with a more contemporary style will usually be spotted in sportier footwear, usually skater-style trainers. In both cases, expect shoes to be paired with brightly coloured stripy socks, or else with so-called 'invisible socks' and a cheeky glimpse of ankle.

OTHER ACCESSORIES

SMARTPHONE

Essential for keeping his Instagram full of countless selfies and for listening to Scott Matthew, Bon Iver, Fleet Foxes...

HEADPHONES

The bigger the better.

SUNGLASSES

Wooden frames are what's hot right now.

BIKE OR SKATEBOARD

Traditional or bohemian types will always go for the bike; more modern guys tend towards skateboards and longboards.

THIS BEARDED LIFESTYLE 2.0 – THE LUMBERSEXUAL APPROACH

If it's a more outdoorsy – by which we mean lumbersexual – look you're after, here are some other items you should consider:

THICK HOODIE

Perfect for when it starts raining when you're out in the woods foraging for mushrooms or silkworms. Try combining it with a check flannel shirt and you're onto a winner.

JEANS

The shabbier the better. After all, good lumbersexual that you are, you're going to be spending half your life hiking through trees, clambering over rocks and surrounded by animals, so you need something comfortable and hard-wearing – yet still flattering.

HIKING BOOTS

Out in the wild a man needs to watch his step, and a pair of tough, high-cut boots are perfect for walking with confidence – and for providing the final touch to your lumberjack look.

ACCESSORIES

WATCH WITH BUILT-IN COMPASS

You'll always know what time it is, it'll help you keep track of when the sun's rising and setting, and the compass will keep you from getting lost.

KNIFE

Whether you need to fight off a fearsome bear, or simply gather some wild mushrooms to eat, a knife will never cease to come in handy.

MAGNIFYING GLASS

Just the ticket for when you're out exploring in the forest and you want to get a closer look at some creepy-crawlies.

CAMERA

Yes, yes, we know your phone takes great photos, but nothing compares to the real thing, especially a vintage analogue camera. Just think how awesome those little birds would look in a Lomo LC-A print!

OTHER USEFUL(ISH) ACCESSORIES

A bit of rope, 'reading' glasses, an illustrated list of poisonous mushrooms...

'BUT REMEMBER – YOU DON'T NEED TO WEAR ALL OF THESE AT THE SAME TIME!'

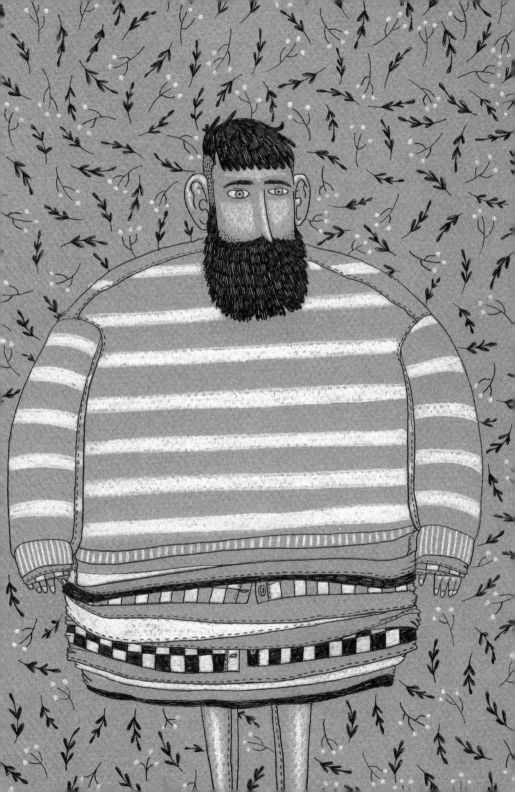

DO BEARDS HAVE MORE FUN?

*Rumour has it that having a beard improves
a man's sex life – but is it just a myth?*

Nobody who's reached this part of the book could possibly deny that today's world is experiencing a veritable beard boom. A golden age for facial hair has dawned over the last few years, and now every hairy-faced man is enjoying his moment in the sun.

The fact is, beards are cool now. Over the last few chapters we've seen how, throughout history, beards have been said to be a sign of wisdom and strength, and those who sport them exalted and praised. Much the same thing is now happening today too – bar a couple of slight differences, of course.

After enduring several eras in which having facial hair meant you were considered little better than a tramp, the humble beard is no longer something to be ashamed of. Quite the opposite, in fact – for now it seems that having a beard hugely increases your sex appeal.

Hey, don't look at us! It's not just wishful thinking: a study carried out at the University of New South Wales – which we'll look at in more detail in the next chapter – found that men with ten days' worth of beard growth were considered most attractive.

One possible sociological reason for why bearded men are now getting more sexual attention could be that they represent a drastic change for the male aesthetic. Not so long ago, the metrosexual look was the order of the day, which meant banishing almost all body hair. Now, however, the ideal man still takes care of his appearance, but aims for a more natural, virile and masculine look – and that means the hairier the better.

But remember – we might be getting all the action, but rest assured that we still get nervous on first dates!

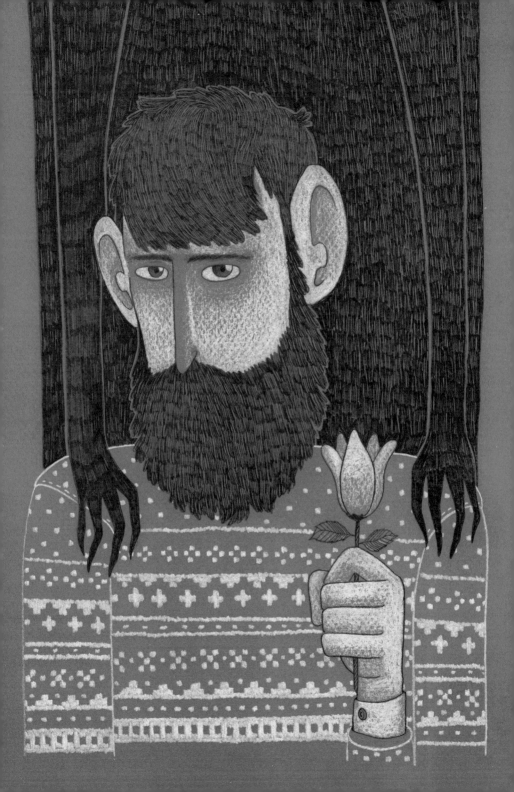

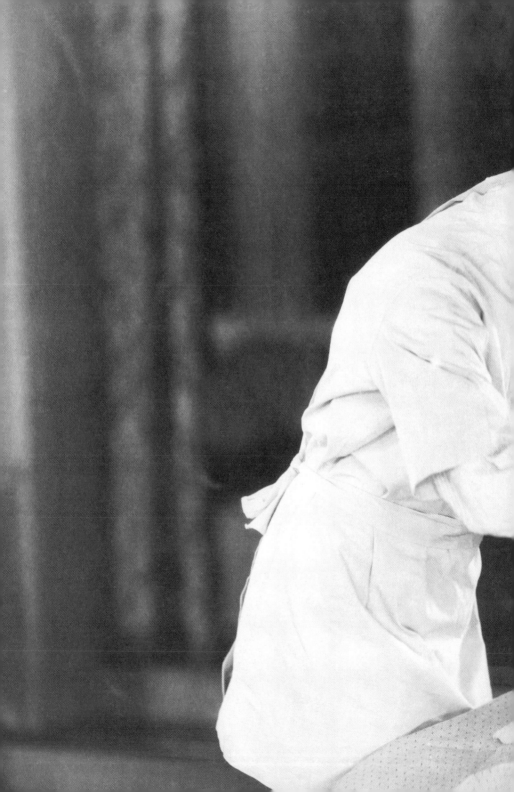

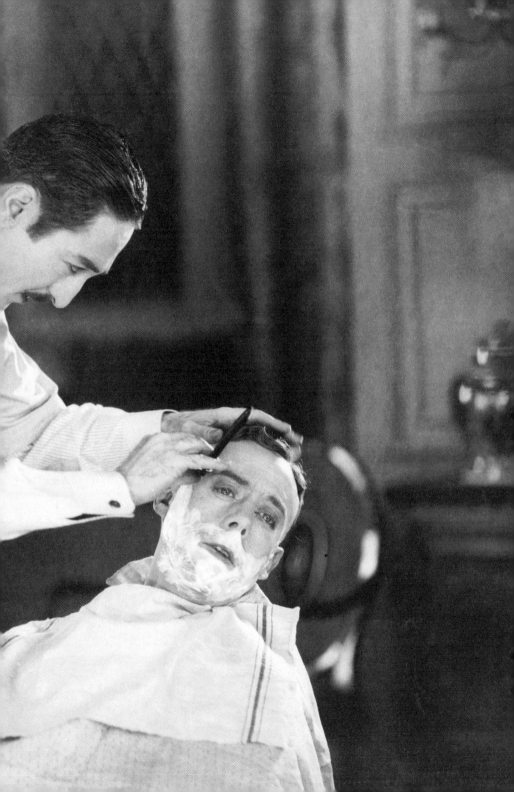

DOES SIZE MATTER?

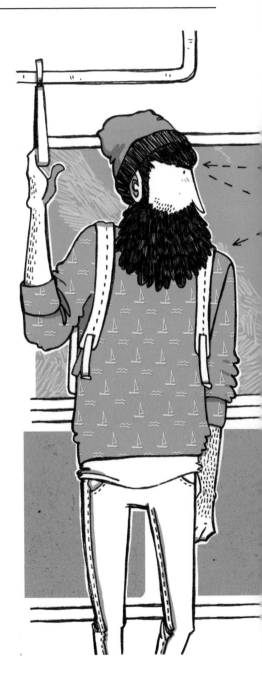

If there are two things the human race simply can't help doing, it's envying and criticising others – and the bearded among us are no exception. In fact, I'd even go so far as to say we're worse than most.

We've all come across the idea that a man's car is an expression of his insecurities regarding the size of his, ahem, manhood. A guy with a big, powerful car is therefore said to be compensating for what he's lacking down below. Now you can agree or disagree with this theory, but there's no doubt that we do tend to believe that size matters more than anything else. We want it all and more besides – end of story.

When it comes to bearded men, the flaws inherent to our humanity combine with those inherent to our... well, beardedness. Within us, mankind's innate tendency to envy combines with the bearded man's pride, and results in a constant, puerile desire to beat our fellow man in the facial hair stakes.

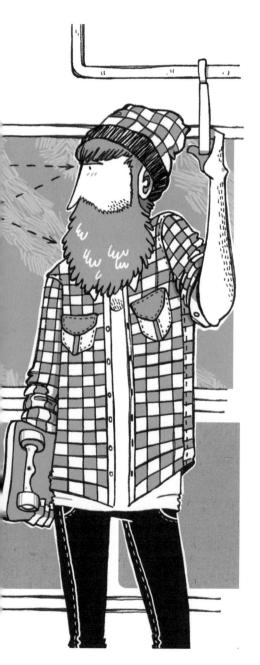

When two bearded men meet – in the street, on the bus, at work – something akin to nuclear fusion (albeit on a smaller scale) takes place. The piercing gaze of each at the other's beard sears through the air, penetrating right the way through to the hair's very roots.

Within a matter of seconds, we'll have analysed not only the products used, but the density, the texture, the pigmentation, the ends and (most importantly) the length of the rival beard. Like two lionesses out on the savannah, we hold one another's gaze – the encounter taking place in slow motion while everything around us moves at double speed to enhance the drama of the moment.

In short, if we really had to answer the question with which we began this section, we would say only one thing:

'A beard should not be measured in centimetres, but in months.'

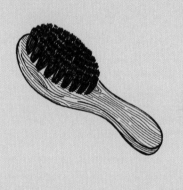

05.

THE MAN
BEHIND
THE BEARD

Facial hair plays two distinct roles:
a metaphysical one,
and an aesthetic one

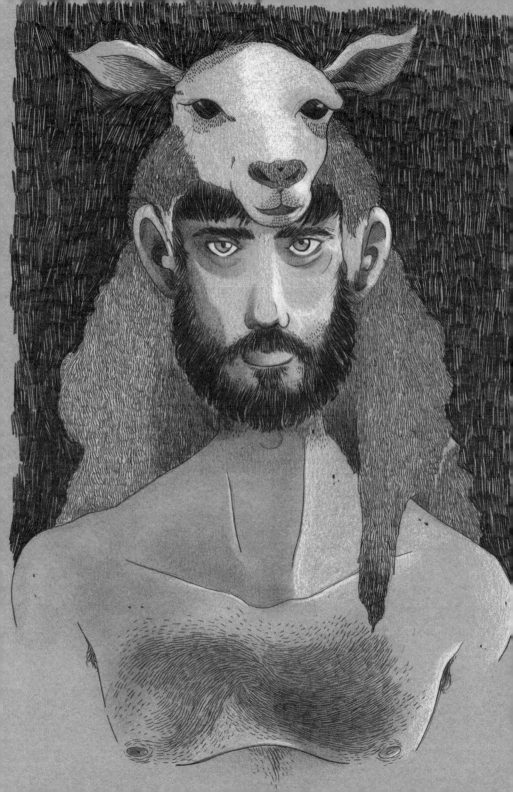

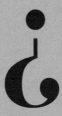

WHAT'S GOING ON
BEHIND THAT BEARD?

Now that we've reached this point in the book – a book which does not purport to be any kind of philosophical or scientific paper on the subject of beards – I think we can say with assurance that facial hair plays two very distinct roles: a metaphysical one, and an aesthetic one.

We began to tackle the first role in the early chapters, looking at how the beard has had, continues to have and will go on having religious, cultural and social significance.

If we take a look at what's been going on in the trendy neighbourhoods of cities across the world (or just flick back to chapter 2) it's easy to see that a new social fabric is being woven with beards at its centre, its members – like hipsters and lumbersexuals – united by their shared taste and sense of style.

In addition to transforming society, however, beards also have the power to influence many other aspects of our everyday lives: fashion, art, photography, advertising, and so on. Which leads us to facial hair's aesthetic role.

That beards fulfil a superficial function is undeniable; they are a physical attribute, after all. Sometimes people grow them because they want to, sometimes because it's fashionable – and sometimes we men use them the way women use make-up: to hide the things we don't want the world to see, and to make the rest look better.

And although there are accounts of so-called bearded ladies presumed to be sufferers of hypertrichosis – Julia Pastrana, or, more recently, Harnaam Kaur – the beard nevertheless remains an irrefutable hallmark of masculinity, something which several studies have illustrated as manifesting itself in many different ways.

THE BEARD MAKEOVER

Having a beard is not – or shouldn't be – simply a matter of having hair on your face. As we've already discussed, a man has to look after his beard to keep it healthy and looking its best – but it's important to remember that the skin beneath your beard also deserves some TLC.

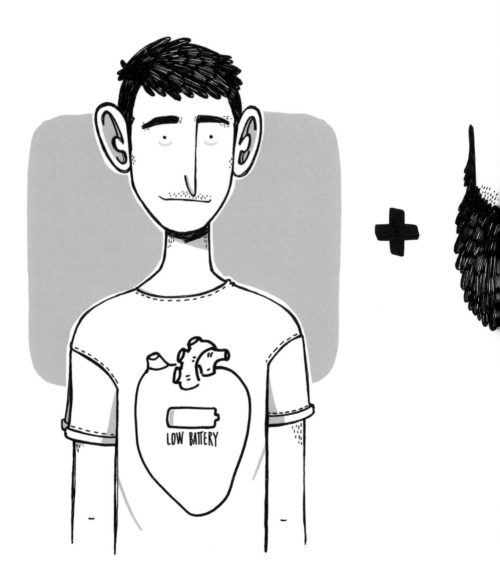

That blanket of hair that covers most of your face can come to your rescue if you're trying to hide or divert attention from any flaws or imperfections, such as spots and scars.

There are also those who use facial hair to enhance their faces, because without it they look strange – babyish and so on. A beard has the power to transform a man's face: to fill it out, to make it look stronger, or to make the man in question look a couple of years older. However, not everybody suits a beard, and certain factors – such as face shape, etc. – should always be taken into account, as we will see a little later on.

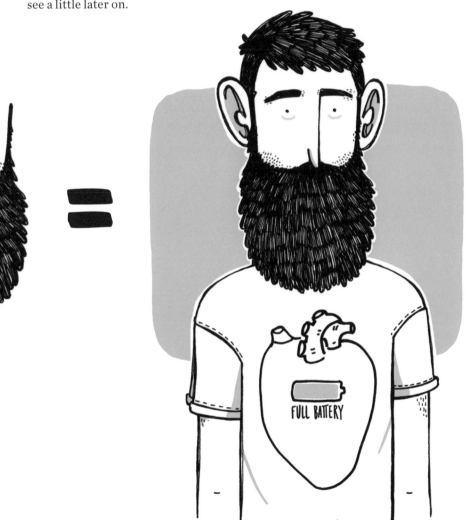

BEARDS AND MASCULINITY

Nowadays, beards are considered an attractive and desirable feature. According to a recent study, facial hair affects perceptions of men's 'socio-sexual' attributes, and women find men with 10 days' worth of beard growth more attractive.

'The beard represents maleness because it is unique to men: it distinguishes one gender from the other. This transforms it into an object of desire, the iconic epitome of masculinity and virility – a sign of beauty and desirability.'

This is what Javier Hirschfeld wrote in his accompanying dossier to the exhibition he commissioned entitled *To shave or not to shave.*

The findings speak for themselves: a study conducted at the University of New South Wales by scientists Barnaby Dixson and Robert Brooks, published in the journal *Evolution & Human Behavior*, found that facial hair affects people's perceptions of men's 'socio-sexual' attributes.

The scientists analysed the reactions of 351 women and 177 heterosexual men upon seeing photographs of 10 different men at four stages of beard growth: clean-shaven; with five days' worth of growth; with 10 days' worth of growth; and finally with a full beard

The results revealed that for the participating women, a medium beard – 10 days' worth of growth – proved the most popular. However, it was the men with full beards that the participants perceived as having the best parenting skills and being most capable of protecting their families.

Though no scientific conclusion was reached to explain the female participants' responses, Dixson and Brooks believe it may be because facial hair helps to make men appear more masculine and more mature.

Meanwhile, another study – carried out by psychologists at Northumbria University and published in *Personality and Individual Differences* – found that clean-shaven men were deemed to possess fewest masculine attributes and to be the least aggressive.

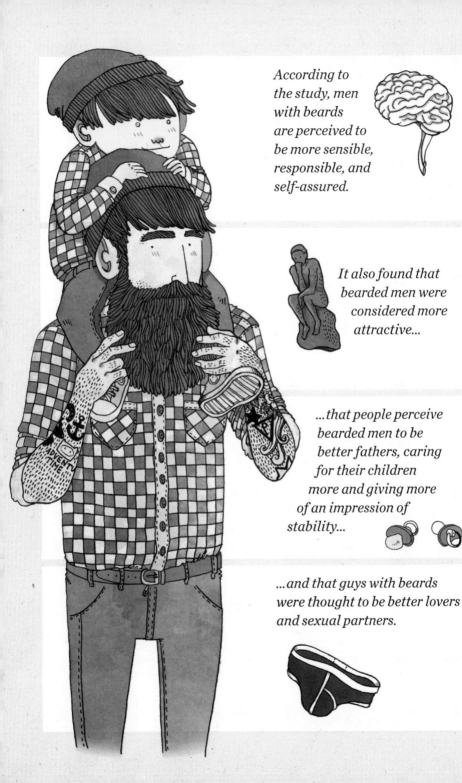

According to the study, men with beards are perceived to be more sensible, responsible, and self-assured.

It also found that bearded men were considered more attractive...

...that people perceive bearded men to be better fathers, caring for their children more and giving more of an impression of stability...

...and that guys with beards were thought to be better lovers and sexual partners.

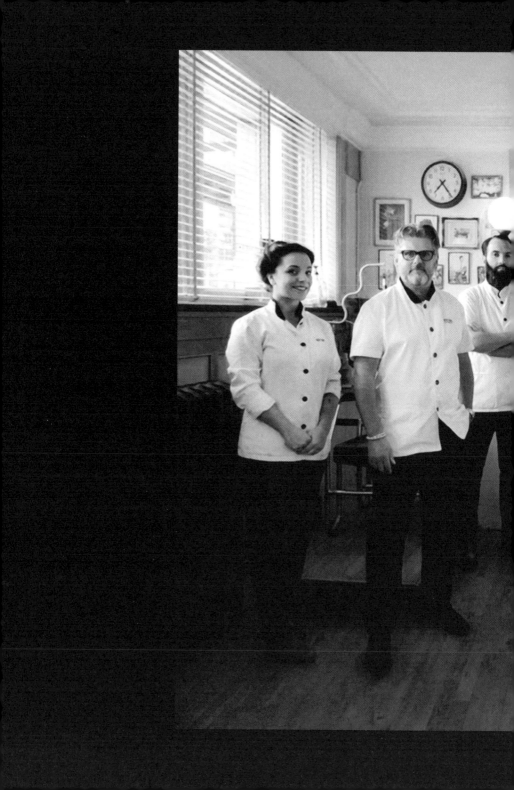

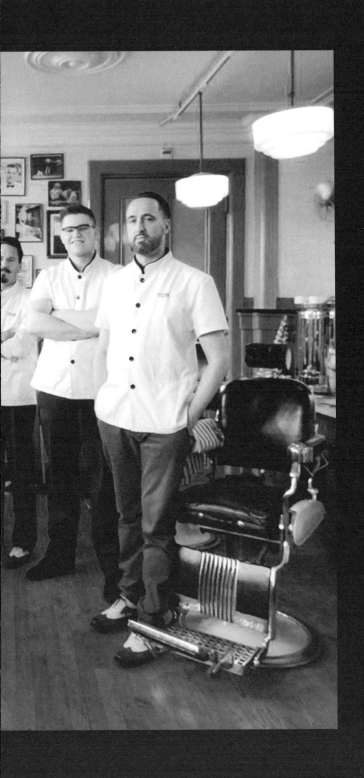

SAYING GOODBYE TO YOUR BEARD

>>> TO <<<

SHAVING

When you actively decide to grow your beard, you form a kind of emotional attachment to it over time. It becomes a part of you, it's with you everywhere you go, bearing witness to everything you do. As a result, if one day you decide to get rid of your furry friend, you might find the experience much more difficult and unpleasant than you might have expected...

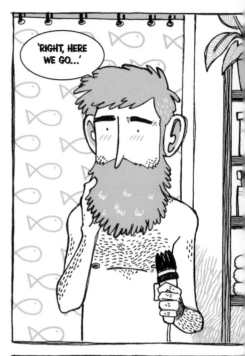

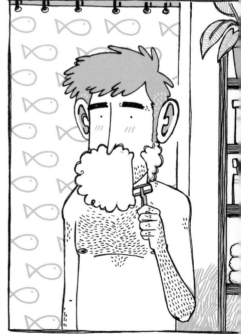

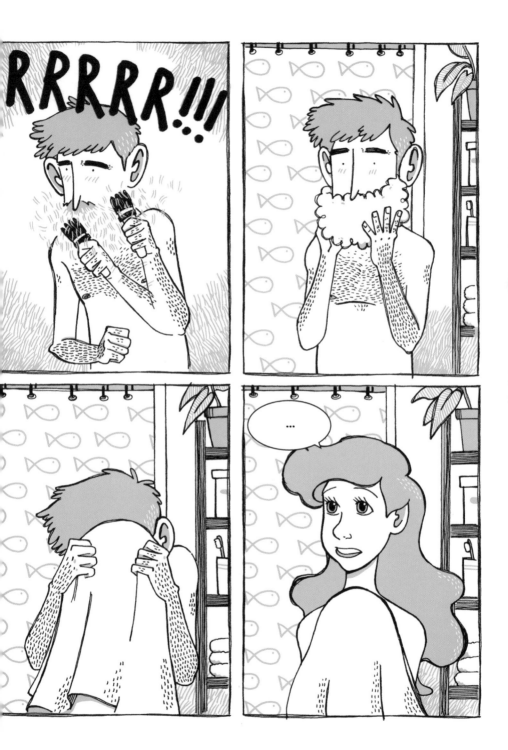

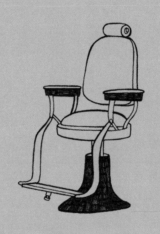

06.

THE WHO'S WHO OF FAMOUS BEARDS

The simple pleasure of growing and looking after one's facial hair is something anyone can fall for

'AUSTRALIAN BAND THE BEARDS FAMOUSLY SANG THAT IF YOUR DAD DOESN'T HAVE A BEARD, YOU'VE GOT TWO MUMS. SO THERE YOU HAVE IT!'

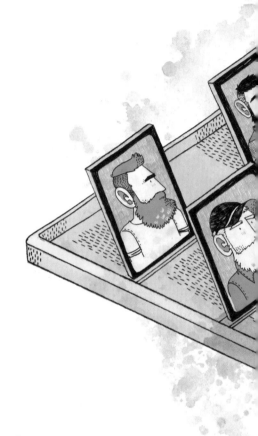

While it's undeniable that everyone seems to be jumping on the beard bandwagon these days, the truth is that there aren't as many celebrities (both past and present) with facial hair as you might think.

Over the next few pages, we've got a selection of photos of some of the most recognizable beards from various fields – music, philosophy, art and cinema – plus some modern-day figures who've been setting a top-notch example when it comes to facial hair.

Now this, really, is nothing more than a brief introduction to a few individuals from past and present who, at some point, decided to grow a beard. We're not claiming to have compiled an exhaustive list here – it's just a little selection of famous bearded faces that we think stand out from the crowd.

And the message we want to convey with this selection is this: that beards are universal and ubiquitous, and that the simple pleasure of growing and looking after one's facial hair is something anyone can fall for.

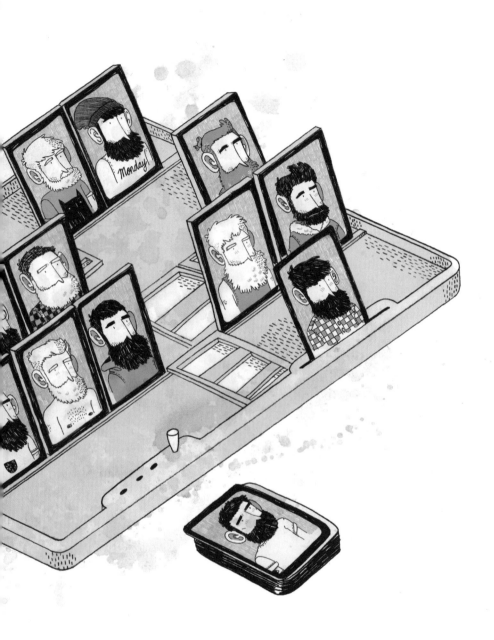

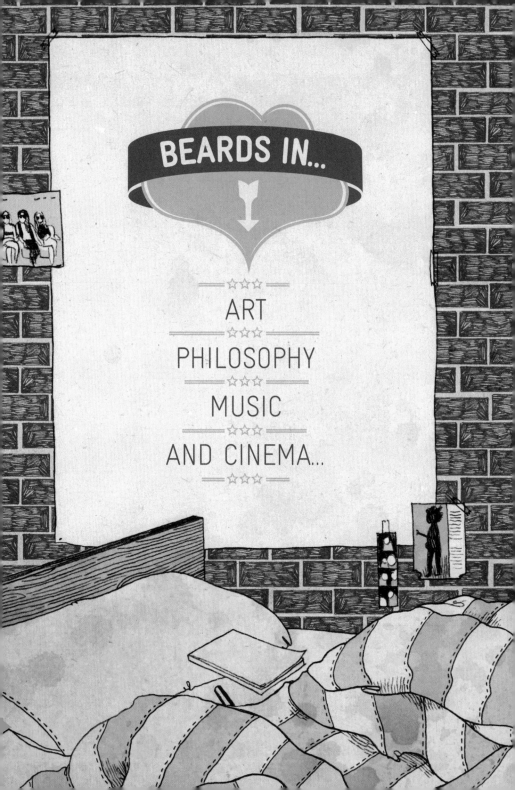

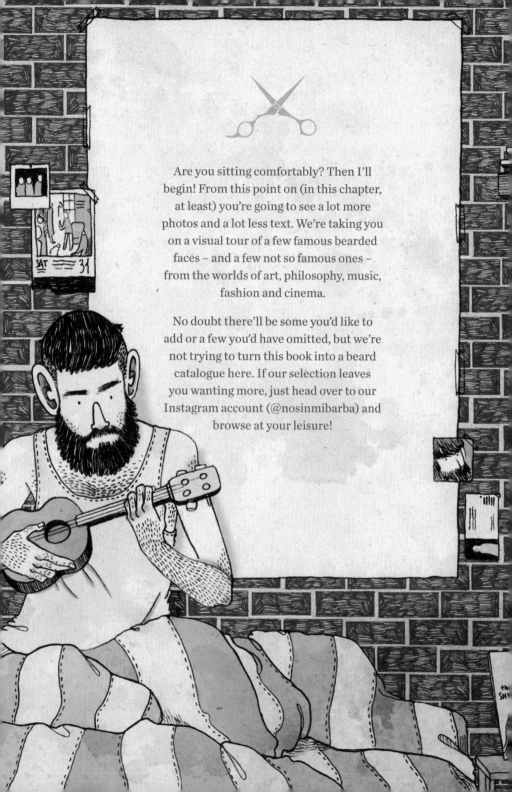

Are you sitting comfortably? Then I'll begin! From this point on (in this chapter, at least) you're going to see a lot more photos and a lot less text. We're taking you on a visual tour of a few famous bearded faces – and a few not so famous ones – from the worlds of art, philosophy, music, fashion and cinema.

No doubt there'll be some you'd like to add or a few you'd have omitted, but we're not trying to turn this book into a beard catalogue here. If our selection leaves you wanting more, just head over to our Instagram account (@nosinmibarba) and browse at your leisure!

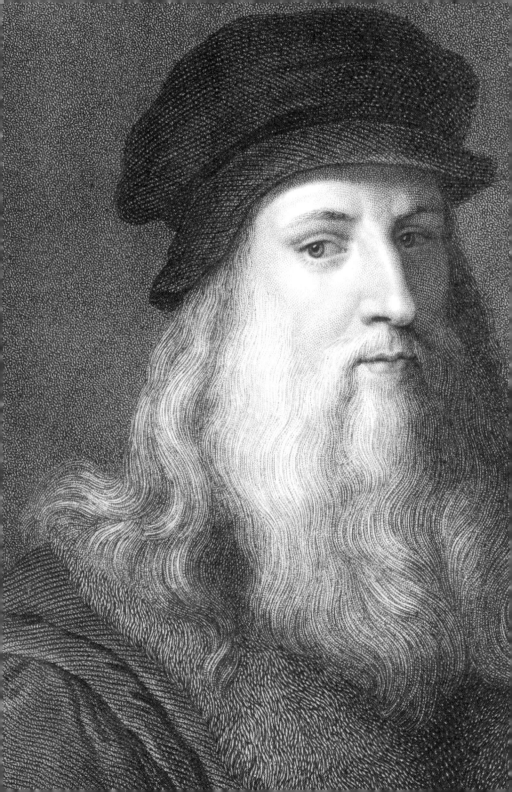

BEARDS IN ART

'IS THERE ANY BEARD IN THE ART WORLD MORE FAMOUS AND MORE UTTERLY RENAISSANCE THAN THAT OF THE MAN WHO BROUGHT US THE MONA LISA, LEONARDO DA VINCI?'

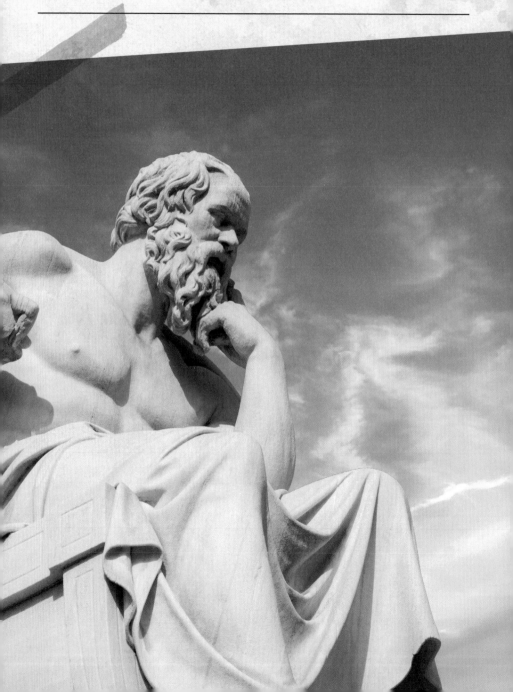

BEARDS IN PHILOSOPHY

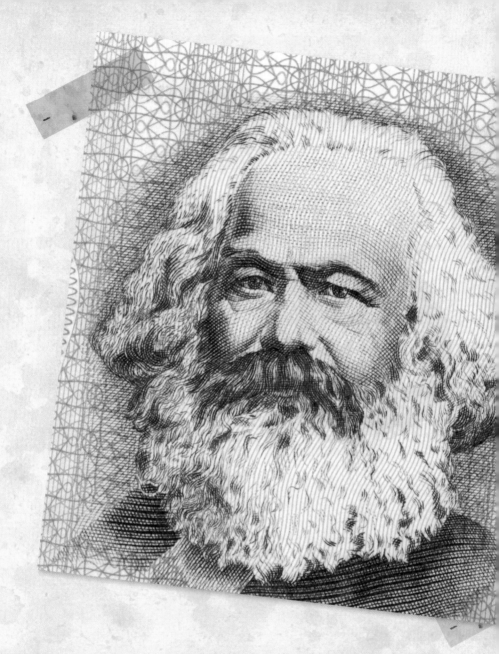

'THE WORLD OF PHILOSOPHY HAS LONG BEEN THE SOURCE OF MANY GREAT BEARDS, FROM SOCRATES RIGHT THROUGH TO KARL MARX.'

BEARDS
IN MUSIC

'BEARDS HAVE ALWAYS LED THE WAY IN MUSIC, TOO - JUST ASK HAIRY LEGENDS LIKE ZZ TOP OR CHET FAKER.'

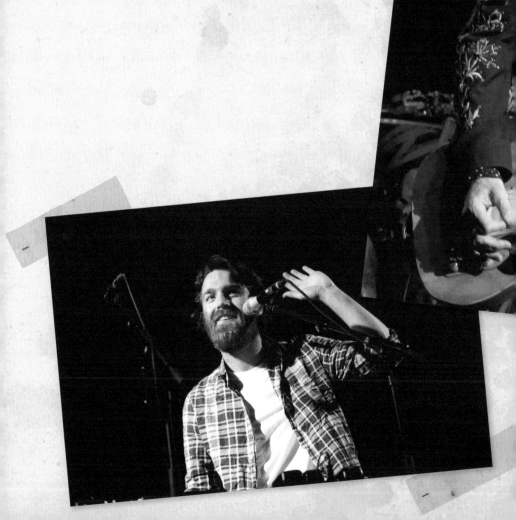

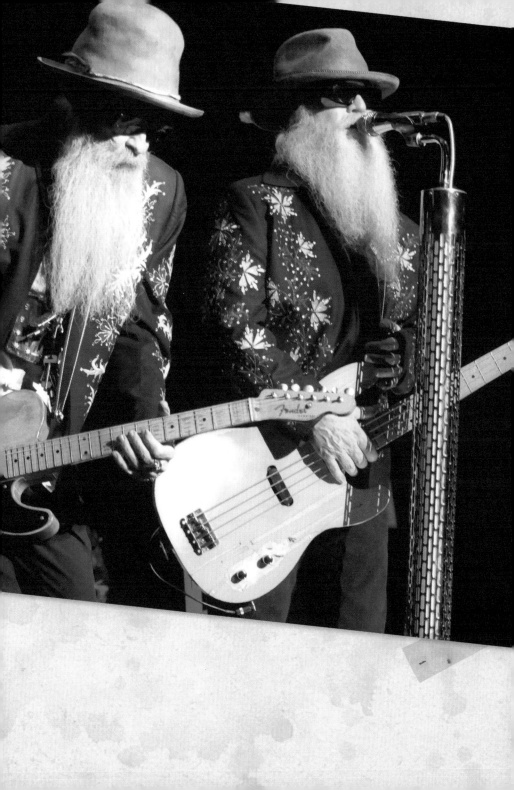

BEARDS
IN FASHION

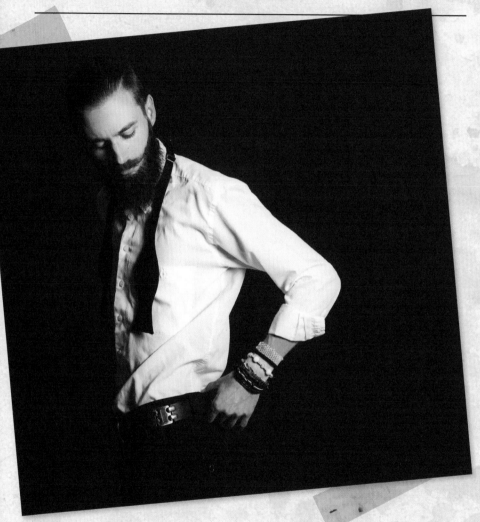

'BEARDS ALSO HAVE THEIR PART TO PLAY IN THE WORLD OF FASHION, AND IN THE LAST FEW YEARS, MORE AND MORE BEARDS HAVE BEEN CROPPING UP ON THE CATWALK.'

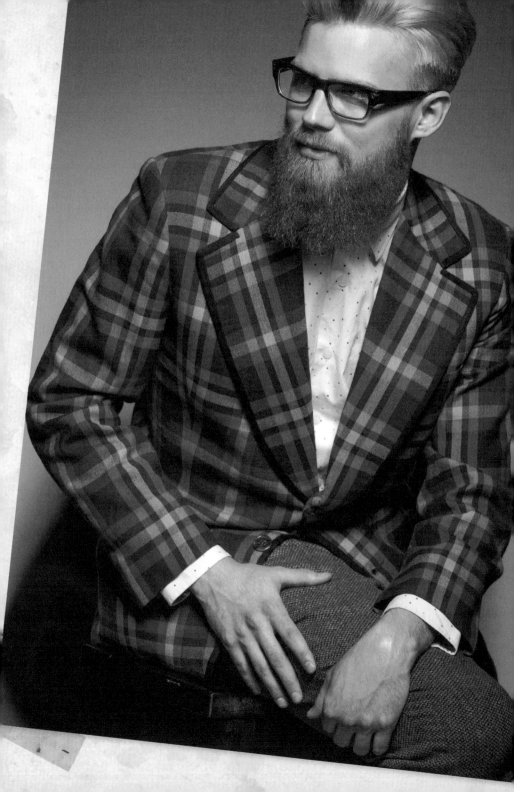

BEARDS
IN FASHION

'AS WE'VE SEEN, BEARDS AND TATTOOS ARE THE PERFECT COMBINATION – AS DEMONSTRATED BY HIPSTER MODEL RICKI HALL.'

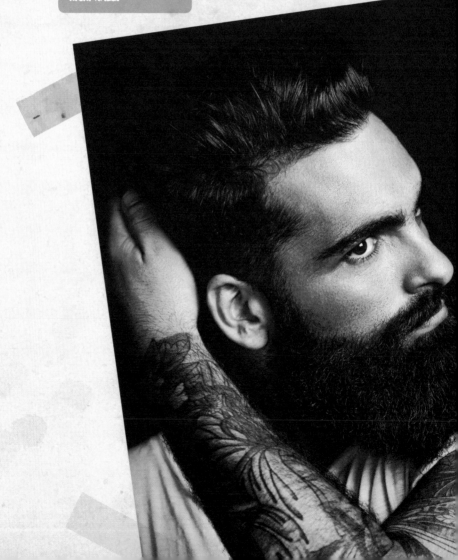

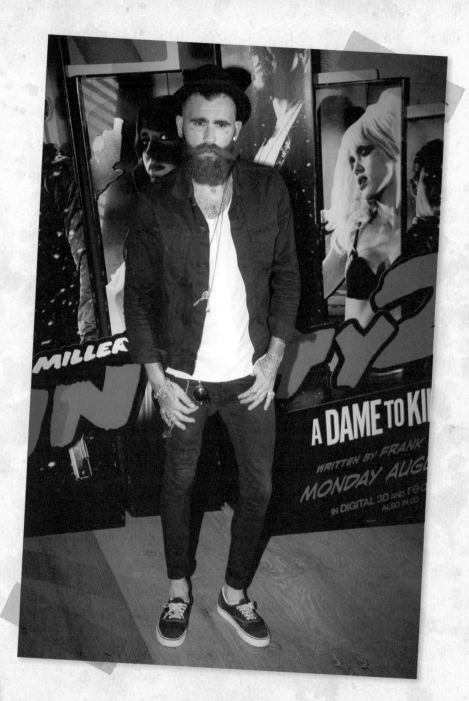

BEARDS
IN FASHION

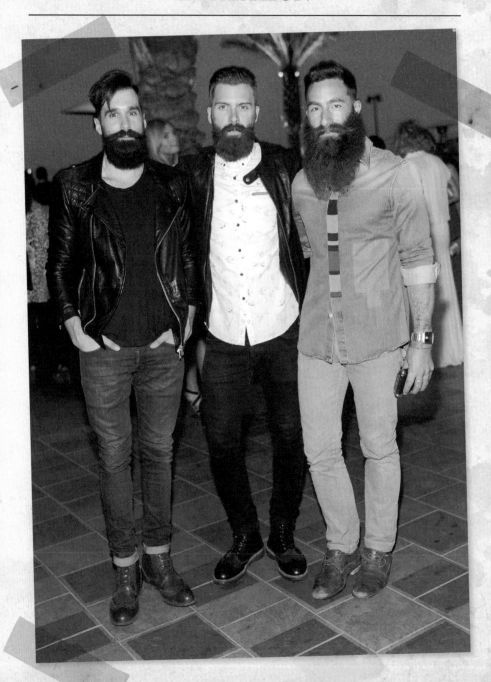

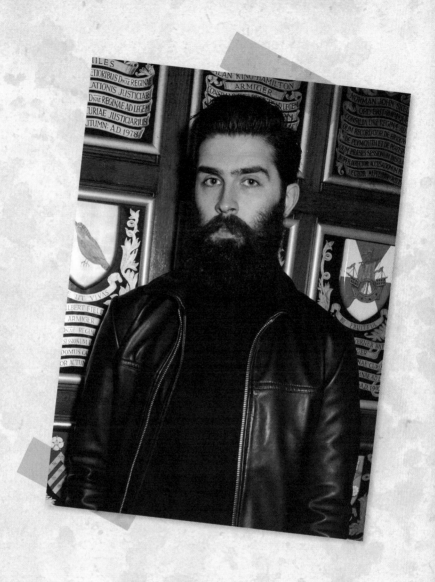

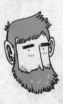

'ON THE LEFT WE HAVE THE BEARDED TRIUMVIRATE OF LUKE DITELLA, LEVI STOCKE AND JIMMY NIGGLES; AND ON THE RIGHT, CHRIS JOHN MILLINGTON.'

BEARDS
IN CINEMA

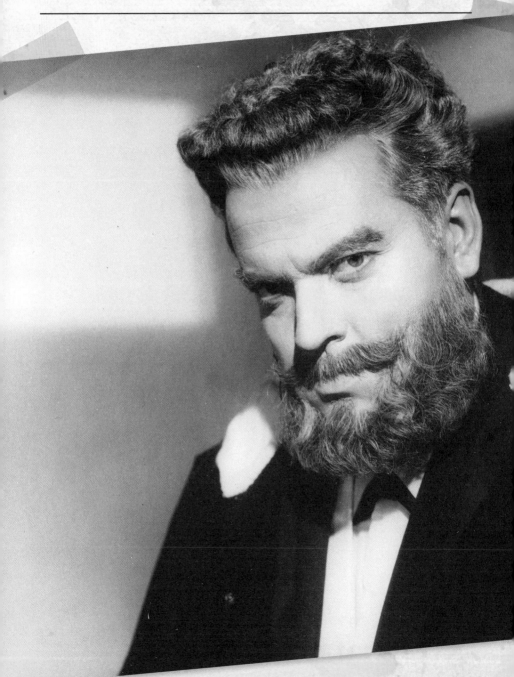

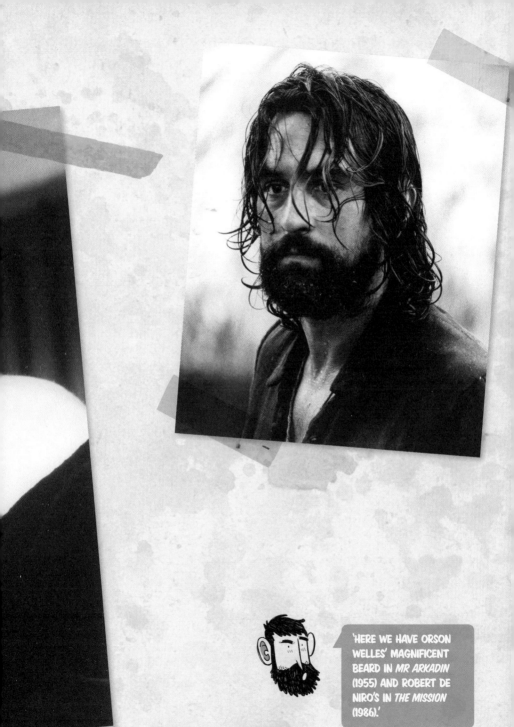

'HERE WE HAVE ORSON WELLES' MAGNIFICENT BEARD IN *MR ARKADIN* (1955) AND ROBERT DE NIRO'S IN *THE MISSION* (1986).'

BEARDS
IN CINEMA

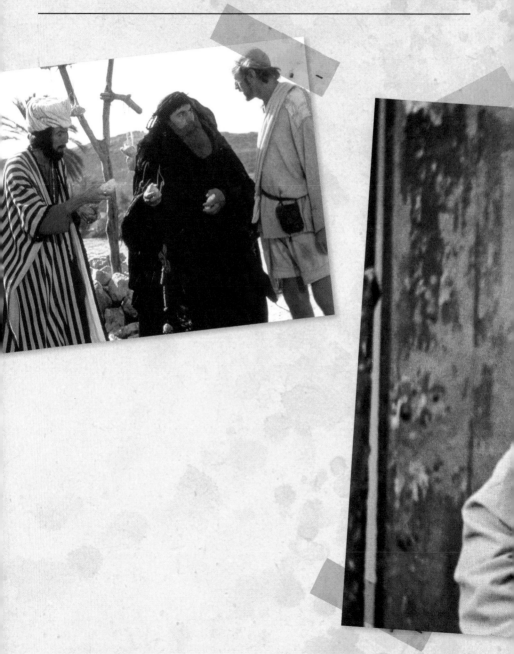

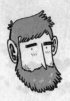

ERIC IDLE, TERRY JONES AND GRAHAM CHAPMAN ALL SPORT VARYING DEGREES OF FACIAL HAIR IN MONTY PYTHON'S *LIFE OF BRIAN* AND 1973 SAW AL PACINO TRANSFORM INTO A HIPSTER COP IN *SERPICO*.

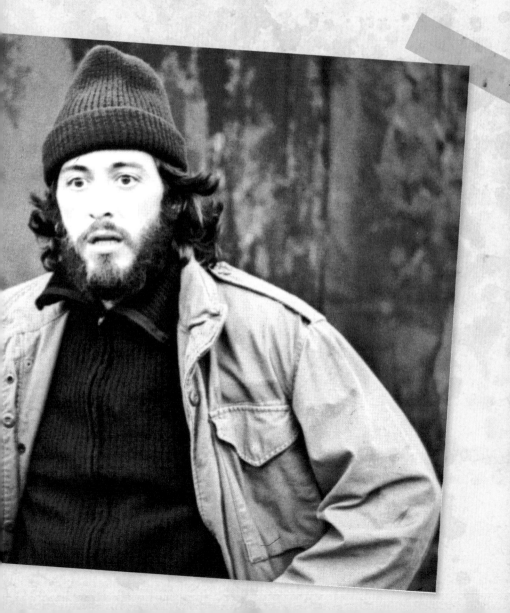

BEARDS
IN CINEMA

'AND IF THERE'S ONE 21ST CENTURY MOVIE BEARD WE ALL KNOW AND LOVE, IT'S BILL MURRAY'S IN *THE LIFE AQUATIC WITH STEVE ZISSOU* - ONE OF HIS MANY TURNS IN WES ANDERSON'S CINEMATIC OEUVRE.'

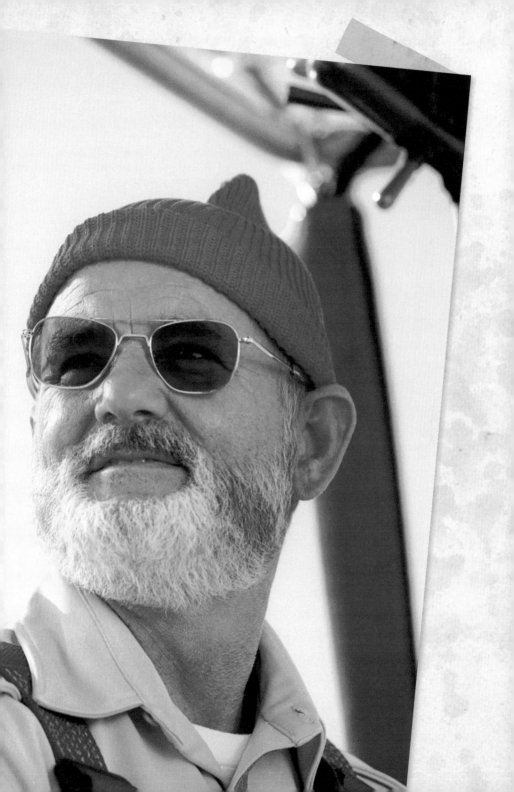

BEARDS
IN CINEMA

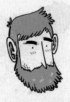

'HERE WE HAVE KIRK DOUGLAS IN *ULYSSES* (1954). NOW
I KNOW IT MIGHT SEEM LIKE HE'S ABOUT TO SHAVE OFF
HIS BEARD, BUT IN FACT HE'S JUST STUFFING HIS FACE
WITH RICOTTA CHEESE...'

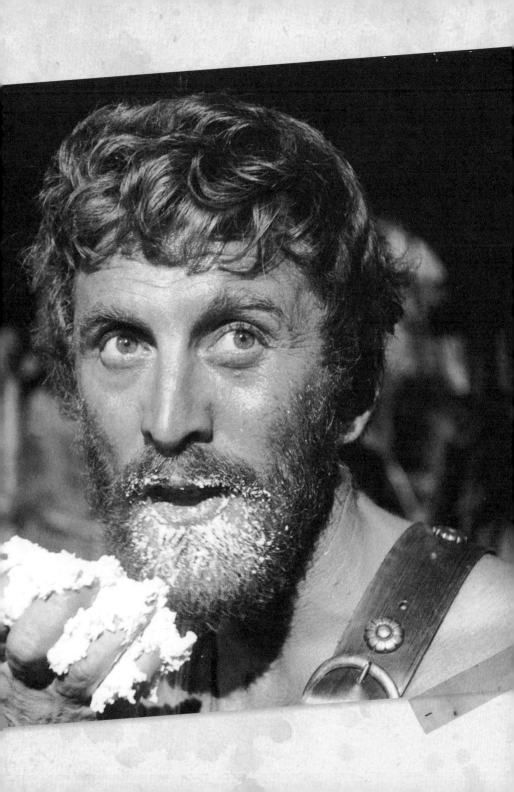

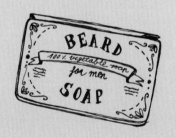

07.

TIPS AND TRICKS FOR THE BEARDED MAN

The beard's rise to stardom is showing no signs of slowing. But growing a beard properly takes time, effort, and a great deal of care

'GRAB A PEN AND PAPER – OR YOUR PHONE, WHICHEVER YOU PREFER – AND SCRIBBLE DOWN THESE IMPORTANT BITS OF BEARD ADVICE.'

The beard's rise to stardom is showing no signs of slowing. On the contrary: be it for fashion reasons or personal ones, more and more guys are choosing to grow their facial hair. But doing it properly is something which takes time, effort, and a great deal of care.

Despite the growing number of men looking for it, the information available about how to look after beards – how to keep them healthy, encourage growth, or which products to use – seems to be patchy at best and, at worst, almost non-existent.

As we saw in chapter 3, this golden age for facial hair has led to both a revival for barbers and a huge rise in the training available for those wanting to become one. Yet in spite of this, no one out there seems to be giving anyone any advice about the basic staples of beard care.

Over the next few pages, we've tried to create a kind of beard manual, divided into three key sections: looking after your beard; how to encourage it to grow; and how to condition it using special beard oils. Please don't think we're trying to lecture you though! Every person, beard and skin type needs different things, but hopefully we can at least offer you a good basic guide – for newcomers and veterans alike.

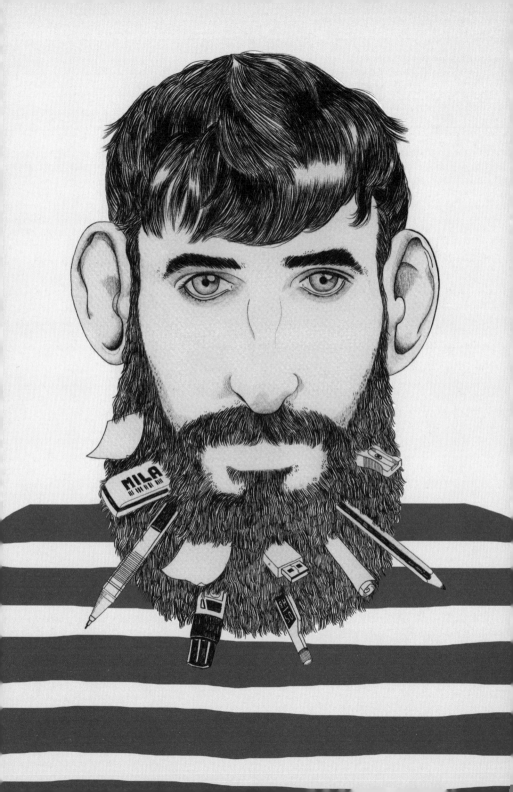

THE THREE BASIC PRINCIPLES OF BEARD CARE

Having – and, more importantly, maintaining – a beard is no mean feat. To a certain extent, whether it grows or not is a question of pure genetics, though other factors can play their part too. But if you've already grown one, and what you want now is to look after it, here are three steps you should incorporate into your daily routine: hygiene, hydration and styling.

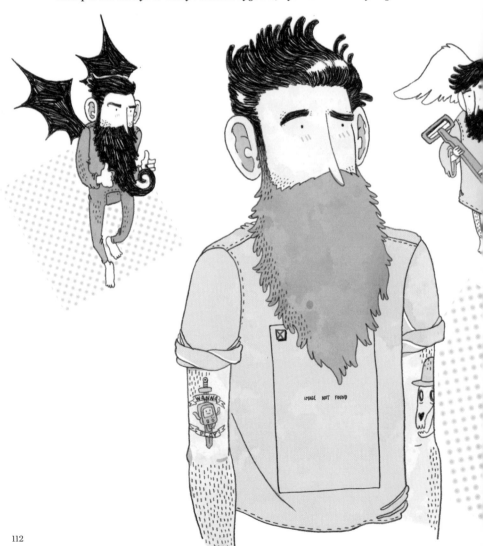

HY GIENE

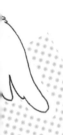

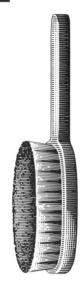

It may seem obvious, but I assure you, it isn't to everyone. Just as you wash other parts of your body daily – face, hands, intimate areas... – so you should treat your beard in exactly the same way. It's exposed to numerous external substances (smoke, bits of food, and so on) which, as well as making your facial hair dirty, can also damage it, while the skin beneath can be prone to developing impurities.

This is why hygiene is such an important part of caring for your beard and the skin underneath it, and why soaps specifically designed for both – be they chemically formulated or 100% natural – should be a staple in the bathroom cabinet of any bearded man.

These soaps work more effectively when your pores are open, so we recommend using them whilst taking a nice, hot shower.

HY DRA TION

As we've already mentioned, growing a beard can make your skin very dry, which can cause it to become sore and flaky. Not only that, but the hair itself feels the effects of dryness too, which is why regular hydration is so very important.

In the third section of this chapter we'll explain what beard oils are and how best to apply them to ensure maximum hydration for our furry friends.

There are other products besides oils which are also designed to hydrate your beard, such as balms. The texture of these beard balms is more like a wax, and you apply them by rubbing a little between your hands and then smoothing it throughout your beard.

Remember, too, that because they are designed to clean and to remove impurities, all beard soaps tend to be astringent, which means they can leave the hair dry, wiry and frizzy. This is why it's so important to hydrate your beard as much as possible, and balms and oils are both a great way to do so.

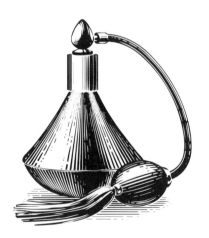

STY LI NG

Shaping and styling a beard isn't as easy as you might think. Though we might want to handle it all ourselves, in my opinion it's essential to seek the assistance of a barber. Once your beard reaches a certain length, it needs more than just the odd trim; taming it and shaping it into the style that best suits your face (something we'll look at more later) requires the trained hands of a professional.

Styling isn't just about the final touches, either. It encompasses everything from shaping your beard to trimming the ends (which you can do at home, but be very careful!); and from shaving (we'll take a closer look at this in 'An essential guide to beard growth') to creating the look you're after.

When it comes to trimming your beard, the most important and fundamental point to remember is not to shave it in a straight line where your neck begins, as this can make it look as though you have a double chin. To avoid this, we suggest following the line of an upside down arc along your neck instead. If you don't want your beard too thick, you can always reduce the volume here too.

If what you're looking for is a long and luxuriant beard, it's important to shape your sideburns and chin area. This allows you to ensure that your beard remains thicker along your jawline and chin than up by your ears.

When all that's left is to style your beard, use a wide-toothed comb or a toothed brush to detangle any knots, and then switch to a bristle brush (natural or bamboo) to smooth the hair as much as possible and distribute any oil applied throughout your beard.

AN ESSENTIAL GUIDE
TO BEARD GROWTH

The thing about beards is it doesn't matter how much you want one, if your facial hair simply isn't genetically disposed to grow, there's not much you can do about it. So if that's your situation... Sorry, but this section isn't going to be of much interest.

For the rest of you – those of you whose facial hair does grow, but who want to know how to make it longer and healthier – here are some pointers to help you look after your beard and encourage it to grow.

HOW CAN I MAKE MY BEARD GROW?

If there's one word you need to repeat to yourself over and over like a mantra while you wait for your beard to grow, it's PATIENCE (in capitals – the capitals are important). Rome wasn't built in a day, and nor can you expect a thick, bushy beard to grow overnight.

If you're not used to letting your beard grow, it's likely you'll experience some irritation and flakiness after the first couple of weeks of growth. Don't worry – it's totally normal for your skin

to dry out as your hair grows. However, here are a couple of tips to help you cope with this:

01.
Moisturise the dry areas with natural products. We suggest using a beard oil, but if you opt for something else, make sure it doesn't contain alcohol, as this will dry the skin out even more and will sting a great deal.

02.
Man up – it won't last long!

Though your beard won't be terribly long at this point and therefore won't require specific washing, try to avoid conventional shampoos coming into contact with the bearded part of your face – they may contain chemical components which could cause irritation.

When your beard emerges from this stage of dryness and soreness, you'll probably find it looks a bit unkempt.

'IF THE IRRITATION AND FLAKINESS DON'T CLEAR UP, SPEAK TO A DERMATOLOGIST.'

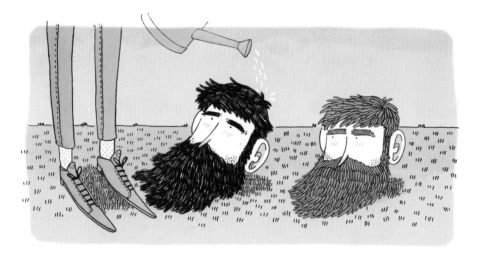

Now's the time to tidy it up, by getting rid of any rebellious hairs growing beyond the desired line of your beard along your neck, cheeks and moustache area. You can do this using a standard razor, an electric one or a Philips laser-guided beard trimmer, or you can ask your barber to give you a once-over with a cut-throat blade. If it's more of a dishevelled castaway look you're after, though, best not to shave at all.

HOW AND WHEREABOUTS SHOULD I SHAVE?

Every so often, razor or shaver in hand, you might find you get rather carried away with the trimming and tidying and cut off a bit more than you meant to. The thing is, you don't really need to shave much at all. Though some guys choose to get rid of all hair anywhere beneath the line of their chin, for example, the truth is this doesn't look very natural; it's much better to start lower, where the straight part of your neck begins.

To groom your moustache, just use a pair of scissors to trim any hairs growing past the line of your top lip. And when you move onto your cheeks, try not to clear too much space – just follow the natural line of your beard, getting rid of any rogue hairs beyond it. Oh, and by the way – that theory that says the more frequently you shave, the faster and thicker the hair will grow? It's a myth, just like all the rest of them.

Once you've decided what kind of beard you want, you just need to wait the time required for it to grow. So if you'd just like a neat, short beard (perfect for those whose employers don't allow anything longer), two or three weeks should suffice. If you're after something bigger, though, we'd recommend you let it grow for a good three months, and after that you can start to tidy it up, trim the ends and shape it into the style you want.

If you're planning on being your own barber, we'd advise you to tackle your beard with scissors rather than a trimmer – you'll have more control, and less opportunity to make a mess of it.

BEARD OIL: THE WHAT, WHY AND HOW

WHAT IS BEARD OIL?

Beard oil is a mixture of various oils which all help to keep your beard healthy and manageable. A base of natural almond or jojoba oil is usually combined with other essential oils – rosemary, for example, or others with strong, pleasant aromas – to nourish and hydrate both your skin and your beard hair, keeping them looking and feeling great.

The quality of the product as a whole will depend on the essential oils combined within it, some of which also have special properties. Once again, rosemary essential oil is a good example of this, as it's been found to stimulate hair growth.

WHY SHOULD I USE BEARD OIL?

Just as you look after your hair by using products specifically designed for that purpose, rather than shower gel, so your beard needs the same level of care.

It faces the elements in much the same way, after all. Wind, cold weather and hard water can all damage facial hair, causing breakage and split ends and leaving it looking rather like a scourer: unkempt and uncared-for.

Here are three simple reasons why you should use beard oil:

01.
IT HYDRATES FACIAL HAIR AND THE SKIN BENEATH IT

Beard oil is an essential product for anyone with a beard because not only does it hydrate your facial hair and help shape it, it also moisturises the skin from which that hair grows. As you probably know by now, beard growth tends to cause skin to dry out, leaving it irritated and flaky – so it's important to keep the whole area hydrated.

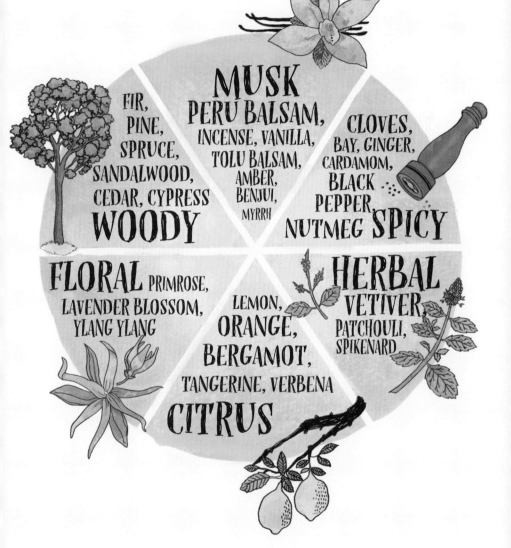

MUSK
PERU BALSAM,
INCENSE, VANILLA,
TOLU BALSAM,
AMBER,
BENJUI,
MYRRH

FIR,
PINE,
SPRUCE,
SANDALWOOD,
CEDAR, CYPRESS
WOODY

CLOVES,
BAY, GINGER,
CARDAMOM,
BLACK
PEPPER,
NUTMEG SPICY

FLORAL PRIMROSE,
LAVENDER BLOSSOM,
YLANG YLANG

HERBAL
VETIVER,
PATCHOULI,
SPIKENARD

LEMON,
ORANGE,
BERGAMOT,
TANGERINE, VERBENA
CITRUS

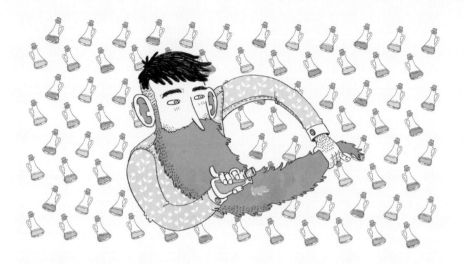

02.
IT PREVENTS BEARD DANDRUFF, SPLIT ENDS AND FACIAL HAIR LOSS

Having a beard isn't as simple as it seems, and there are certain 'hairy' situations you'll want to avoid. The first? Beard dandruff – the result of the flaky skin we talked about earlier. The second is split ends – hairs which have split into two or three tips; and the third is hair loss, caused by facial hair becoming weakened. Beard oil tackles all three problems because it strengthens and hydrates facial hair – along with the added bonus of helping you to shape and style your beard too.

03.
IT KEEPS YOUR BEARD SMELLING GREAT

Thanks to the many essential oils which can be combined to create them, beard oils come in a huge variety of scents for you to choose from: citrus, floral, herbal, spicy, balsamic or woody.

WHEN IS IT BEST TO APPLY BEARD OIL?

By far the best time to apply beard oil is when your pores are at their most open and receptive – which means after taking a shower or washing your face. We really can't emphasise enough just how important hydration is for keeping your beard healthy!

If your beard is particularly dry or coarse, we strongly recommend using beard oil every day, just after giving your facial hair a thorough wash. As for other beard types, though it's not strictly necessary, we'd still recommend a daily dose of oil: it will keep your facial hair stronger and healthier, leaving your beard always looking its best.

HOW DO I APPLY BEARD OIL?

It's dead easy – provided you remember that the idea is not to go around with a beard so full of oil that innocent bystanders are blinded by how shiny it is, or else you'll look like you're greased up for a Turkish wrestling match.

So: just gently massage three or four drops into your beard, and in a matter of moments you'll look a million dollars.

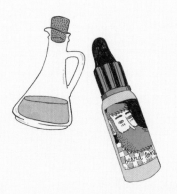

01.

Get three or four drops of oil in your hand

02.

Rub your hands together to cover them both in oil. The heat generated will activate and intensify the oil's aroma.

03.

Massage the oil into your beard and the skin beneath. If your beard is particularly long and thick, we recommend you start on your chin area and try to make the oil stretch right to the tips of your hair.

04.

Shape your beard with your hands or with a special beard brush. Now it should look, feel and smell great!

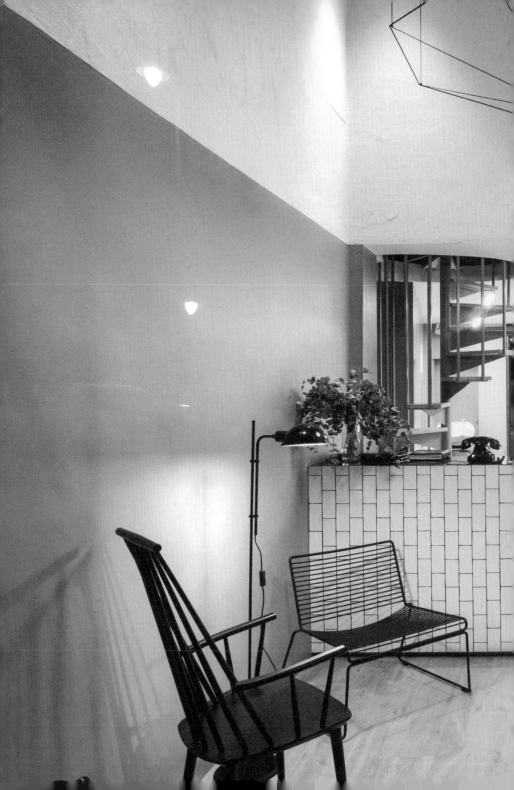

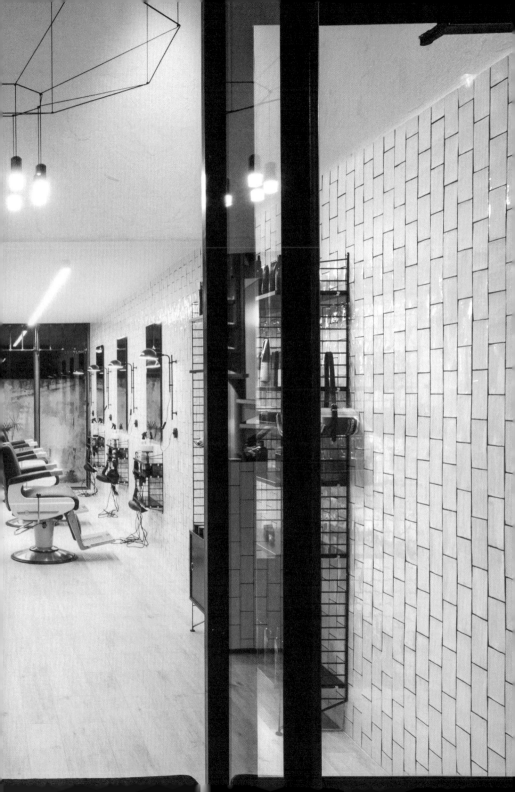

WHICH IS THE RIGHT BEARD FOR MY FACE?

This is one of the questions most frequently asked by guys just starting to grow a beard – a question barbers probably have to answer several times a day.

But before you can find out which beard will suit you best, you have to know what kind of face shape you have. Of course, really there are as many face shapes in the world as there are people, but generally they fall into a few major categories. In this section, we're going to show you the five most common face shapes and how to figure out which one you have – via a quick lesson in stylistic geometry.

First, let's take a few facial measurements – starting with these horizontal ones:

Temple to temple

Cheekbone to cheekbone

Jaw to jaw

Now let's go vertical! Measure the distance from your hairline (in the middle of your forehead) to the tip of your chin, and divide it by 3. Finally, measure the distance from the bottom of your nose (just beneath it, from the top of your moustache) to the tip of your chin once more.

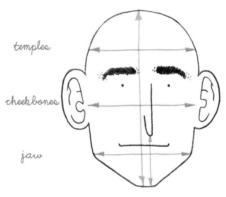

Once you've got all those measurements written down, keep reading to find out the face shape you have and which beard will suit you best:

01.

If the three horizontal measurements you took all came out equal, your face shape is square. If this is the case, your face best suits a fine beard without much volume, which will soften your features. Opt for anything else and you'll only make your face look even more square.

02.
HEART-SHAPED

If the distance between your temples is greater than the distance between your cheekbones, you've got a heart-shaped face. A beard that's nice and thick around the chin area, paired with long sideburns with a bit less volume, will help bulk up the narrow lower part of your face.

03.
ROUND

If the result you got when you divided the distance from your hairline to your chin by 3 is greater than the distance between your chin and the base of your nose, then your face shape is round. The best option for you is a goatee or goatee and moustache combination (sideburns are also a possibility) as this will elongate your face.

04.
LONG

Your face shape is long if the distance between nose and chin is 0.5 cm greater than the hairline-chin distance divided by 3. If you have a long face, you can grow your beard all across your chin, but don't let it get too thick, as this will lengthen your face further.

05.
OVAL

On an oval face, the distance between nose and chin is 0.5 cm shorter than the hairline-chin distance divided by 3. If this is you, count yourself lucky: any beard style suits this kind of face. But don't get too cocky – that doesn't mean you don't still have to look after it!

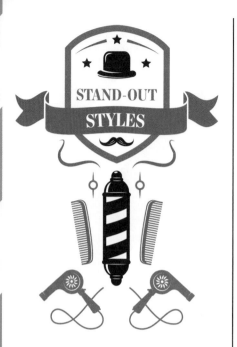

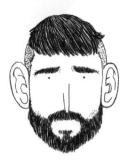

FULL BEARD

Beard, 'tache and sideburns are all connected in this style. Like the Verdi, the full beard is particularly recommended for oval or heart-shaped faces, provided it's not grown too long.

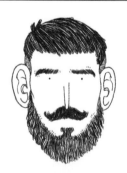

VERDI

This style is all about the stand-alone moustache, totally detached from both beard and sideburns. Recommended for oval or heart-shaped faces (if not grown too long).

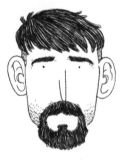

VAN DYKE

Recommended for those with round faces, the Van Dyke features a moustache grown to connect with a goatee (hair only grown on the chin, not along the jaw).

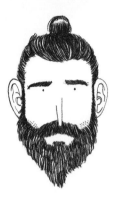

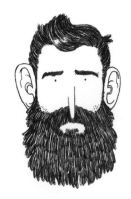

DUCKTAIL

To create this beard, the sideburns are kept short while the hair on the chin area is allowed to grow longer and thicker, shaped into a pointed tip – like a duck's tail. Ideal for oval or heart-shaped faces, though don't let the 'tail' get too long.

RAW

Among the most popular styles of the moment, this look features both beard and moustache grown long, thick and untamed. Though everyone's jumping on the raw bandwagon these days, it's not a style that suits every face – but if yours is an oval shape, go as wild as you like.

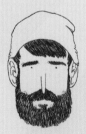

GARIBALDI

Though otherwise very similar to the raw style, the Garibaldi gives the beard a distinctive rounded bottom.

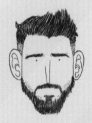

EXTENDED GOATEE

This style is not a million miles away from the ducktail beard. With sideburns starting low and the hair grown longer around the chin area, the extended goatee looks great on heart-shaped faces.

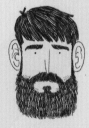

TRIMMED

To create this style, facial hair is thinned to keep it fine, using trimmers or scissors. It works well on long faces as it doesn't add too much volume, and it's great for softening square faces too.

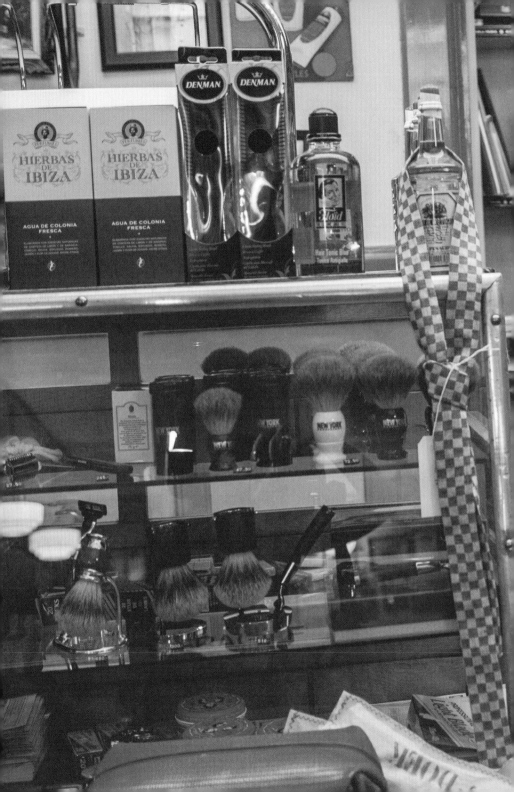

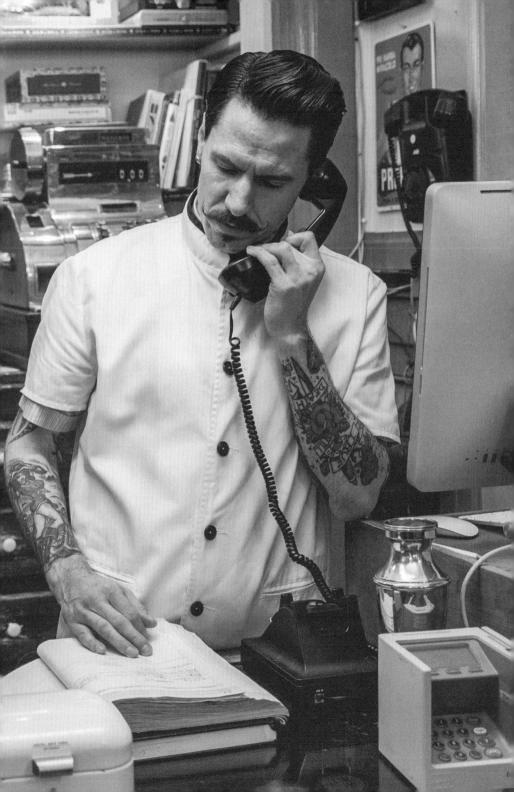

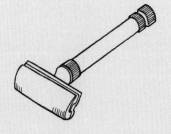

08.

APPENDICES

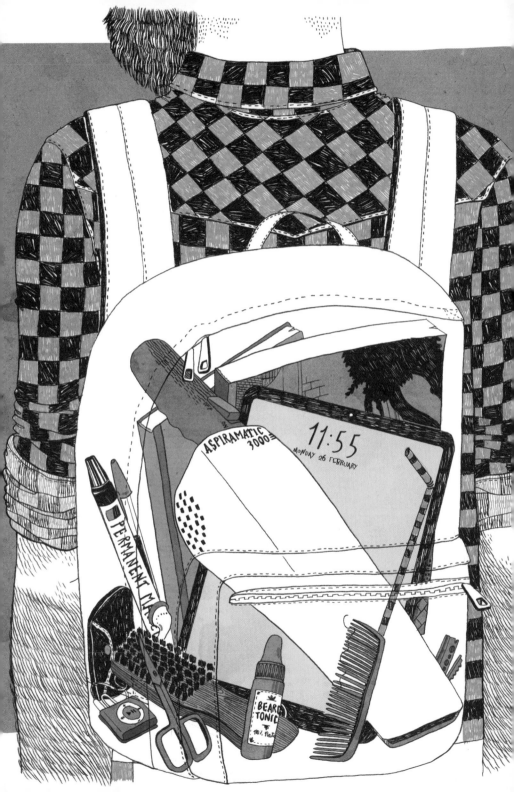

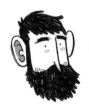

'HAVING AND LOOKING AFTER A BEARD IS A BIG RESPONSIBILITY, BUT THERE ARE LITTLE THINGS YOU CAN DO TO MAKE IT EASIER – AND THAT'S WHERE WE COME IN!'

Throughout these pages, we've stressed the importance of looking after your beard I'd say, oh, only about 804 times. Hopefully we've made it crystal clear that every one of us bearded folk needs to keep our hairy friend washed, hydrated and styled, and that there are hundreds of products out there to help us do just that.

But pampering our beards with special treatments and rituals isn't enough; we also have to keep a close eye on them all throughout the day, to make sure they don't get dirty, that they don't dry out, and so on. In short, living with a beard isn't always easy, and it's a lifestyle that's full of potential enemies: crumbs, wind, cold, cappuccino foam...

This is why it's imperative that any self-respecting beard owner never leave the house without putting together his own personal facial hair survival kit, like the one you can see on the opposite page.

In the rucksack of your standard bearded man, you can expect to find the usual collection of essential items: iPad, iPod, iPhone (or similar non-Apple devices), wallet, keys – plus, of course, a copy of *This Bearded Life*, and a notebook and pen for scribbling down ideas.

But if he's a true facial hair fanatic, he'll also have with him some beard oil, a pair of scissors so he can trim his moustache at a moment's notice, a comb for getting rid of any knots, and a brush to keep his beard looking tidy. And the very pinnacle of preparedness? Carrying around a straw, for having a few beers with his work mates without worrying about getting a foam 'tache, and a handheld hoover, for doing away with any lingering crumbs in his facial hair.

What else do you think should go in our survival kit?

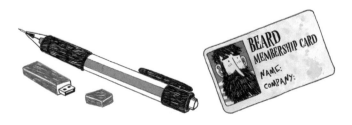

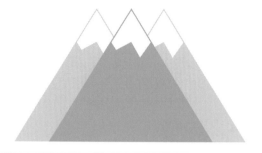

A HAIRY SITUATION

FINALLY! The weekend has arrived and you've decided to make the most of it by going on a little trip with your girlfriend – some well-earned time away from your irritating brother-in-law, your exhausting colleagues and your mother's constant nagging. It's only a couple of days and you're only going to Cuenca, but hey, it's actually much prettier than people say...

Soon enough it's time to start packing for the weekend: in go your sunglasses, driving licence, shampoo – and beard soap, of course. Then you realise you'd better take some beard oil too, or perhaps a balm, and some conditioner;

you'll need your beard comb and brush for detangling and styling as well, not to mention some wax for your moustache, something scented maybe... Before you know it, your rucksack is bursting at the seams and anyone would think you were off on a month-long trek rather than a weekend city break.

To cap it all, you then realise your girlfriend's managed to fit everything she needs into a tiny bag about 23 times smaller than yours – so, naturally, she tells you you're being ridiculous. But what does she know? Your beard deserves the best.

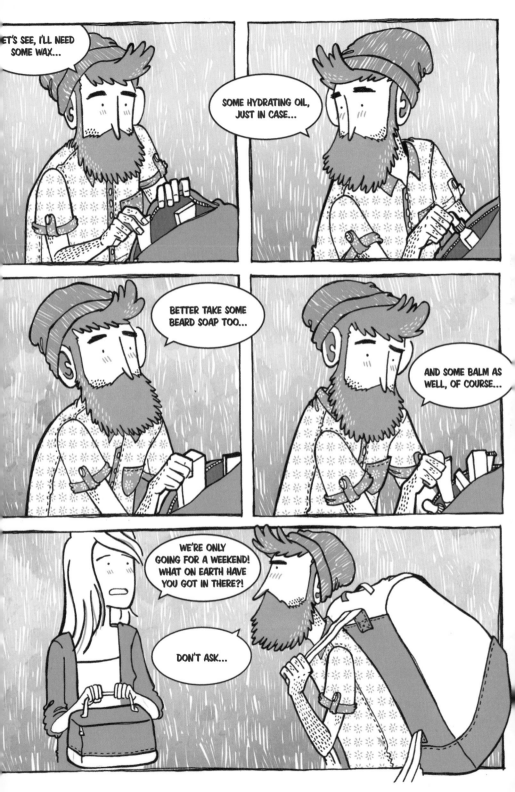

THIS BEARDED LIFE GLOSSARY

*Here you'll find definitions for some of the words we've used in this book,
plus a few others related to all things facial hair*

Aftershave

Cream designed to hydrate and repair your skin after, well, shaving!

Beard

Facial hair which grows on the cheeks, chin and neck, as well as around the lips – generally on men.

Beard density

This term refers to the concentration of facial hair per centimetre squared. The more developed the beard is and the thicker each individual hair is, the greater the beard density.

Brushes

There are many different types of beard brush available, and they vary not only in terms of size and shape, but also in terms of what kind of bristles they have – though generally the bristles will be made either of bamboo or of some other kind of natural material. Brushes are great for ensuring even distribution of oil or balm throughout your beard.

Cheeks

Facial area on which hair grows, connecting sideburns, moustache and chin hair.

Cheek line

This is the line that marks your beard's upper limit on your cheek. The cheek line can be defined using a trimmer or razor, or it can be left to develop naturally.

Chin

Area beneath the lower lip where hair (generally) tends to grow.

Combs

Combs are essential when it comes to shaping and styling your beard. Depending on the size of the comb's teeth, these can be used to untangle knots in your beard (wide-tooth combs) or to simply comb it smooth (fine-tooth combs). You can now also get pocket combs, for beard maintenance on the go, and combs specifically designed for moustache care.

Cut-throat razor

Sharp-bladed tool used by barbers to perform shaving treatments. The blade can usually be changed and replaced, and must be disinfected regularly.

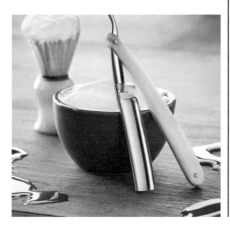

Facial hair

This term can be used to refer either to the beard as a whole or to a single part of it, i.e. your moustache can also be described as 'facial hair'.

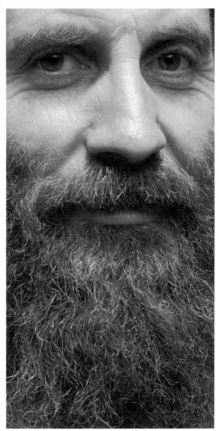

Full beard

Beard style in which hair is grown in all possible facial areas: chin, cheeks, moustache, side burns – the lot.

Goatee

Beard style in which hair is grown exclusively on (and sometimes just beneath) the chin area, generally paired with a moustache.

Moustache

Hair which grows between the base of the nose and the upper lip.

Neck line

This is the line that marks your beard's lower limit across your neck. The neck line can be defined using a trimmer or razor, or it can be left to develop naturally.

Pigment

The substance which gives hair its colour.

Razor blade

Sharp pieces of metal used in safety razors (hence the name) which can be replaced when they become blunt.

Safety razor

This is an alternative to the cut-throat razor, also used by barbers to perform shaving treatments. Classic safety razors are usually made out of stainless steel and have blades which can be changed and replaced. Nowadays, disposable safety razors and electric shavers (not to be confused with trimmers) are also available for the general public to buy and use.

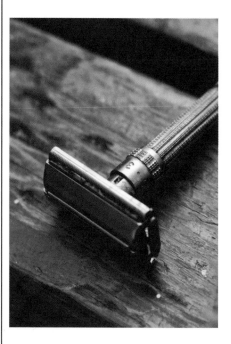

Shaving brush

One of a barber's essential tools, used to help distribute shaving foam evenly across the area to be shaved.

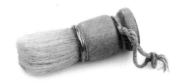

Shaving foam or cream

A product which facilitates a close, irritation-free shave, leaving skin feeling fresh and moisturised.

Shaving mug

Small receptacle used to whip shaving cream into a lather.

Sideburns

This refers to the strips of hair that grow next to your ears, connecting your beard with your hairline.

Texture

The facial hair characteristic which determines whether your beard hair will grow straight or curly.

Trimmers and shaping tools

Electronic devices which allow you to shave, shape and/or trim your facial hair depending on which setting or attachment you use. These are great for creating and maintaining very defined beard styles.

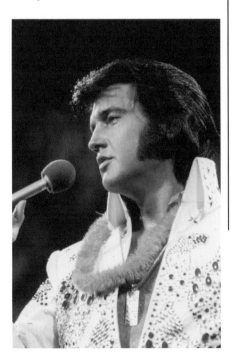

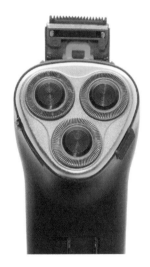

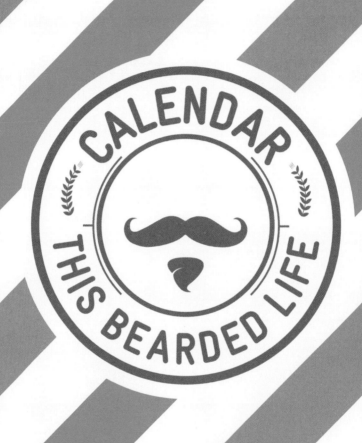

Time doesn't move in the same way for us bearded folk as it does for other mortals. In addition to all the usual daily activities of your average human being, we also have to attend to the crucial task of looking after our beards. And I'm not just talking about washing and moisturising it (though obviously that is of paramount daily importance); I'm talking about long-term care and maintenance.

As discussed earlier, growing a beard is a matter of time (and patience) – which is why we're giving you this helpful calendar, so that you can record all your important facial hair facts and figures (growth, condition, products used, etc.). We've also taken the liberty of including a few notes of our own which we're confident you'll thank us for.

JANUARY
You decide that one of your New Year's resolutions will be to grow your beard. Good for you! Come join the party!

··

FEBRUARY
Your partner buys you lots of beard care products
for Valentine's Day from
www.nosinmibarba.com.

··

MARCH
You're now into your second shaving-free month
and it's starting to yield results. Give the ends a trim
but otherwise, leave it be!

APRIL

At last, your beard is coming along nicely – congratulations! Now it's the barber's turn to give it a little tidy-up, and from now on, you should make an appointment every couple of weeks to keep your beard in check.

JUNE | JULY | AUGUST

All that sun, swimming and salt can dry out and damage your beard, so don't forget to keep your supply of oils and balms to hand. And remember, *This Bearded Life* is full of all the beard care tips and tricks you could possibly need!

OCTOBER | NOVEMBER | DECEMBER

Winter can be tough on your beard, so be sure to take extra special care of it during these chilly months. Keeping it nice and hydrated will ensure it stays strong and healthy, even in the face of cold, blustery weather.

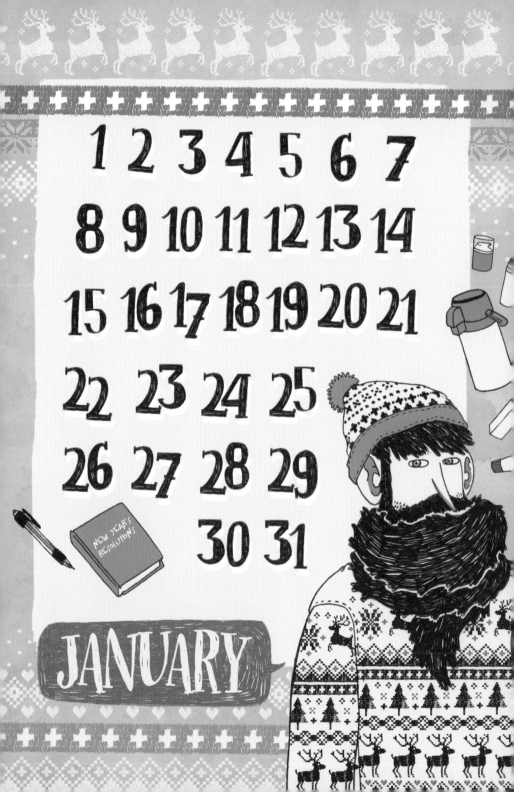

JANUARY

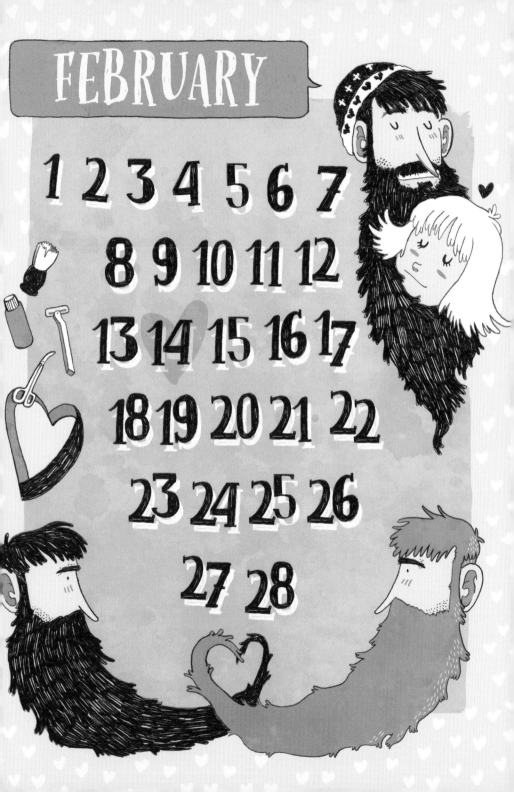

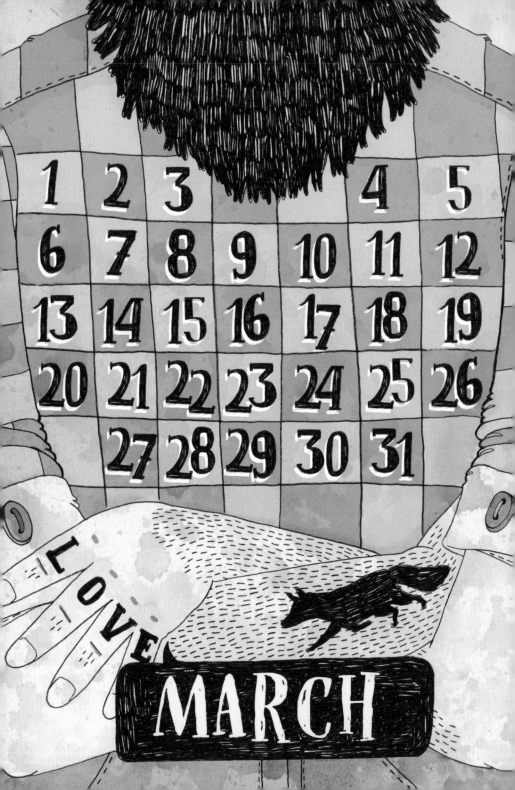

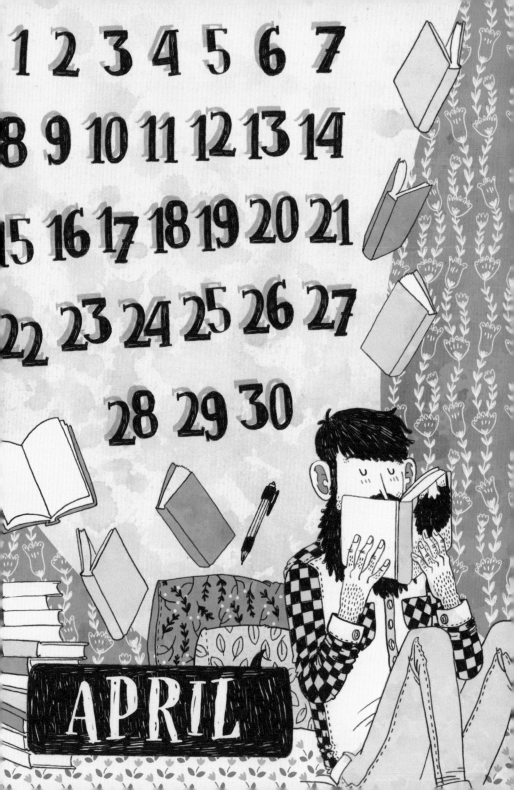

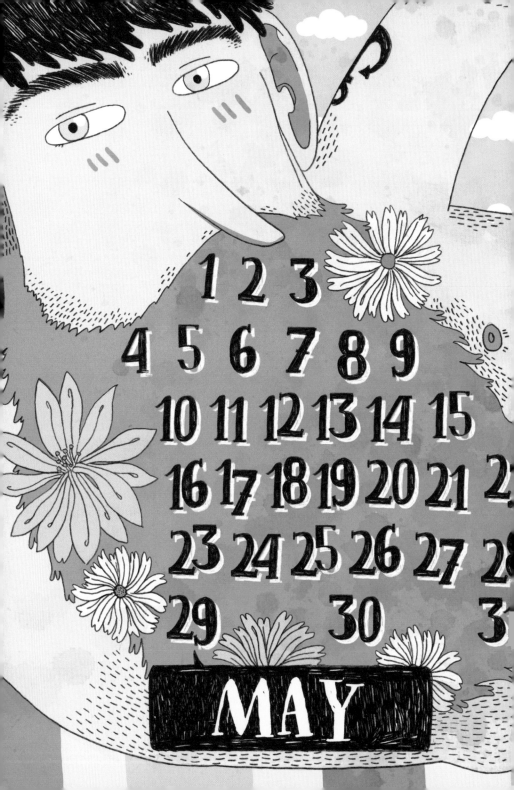

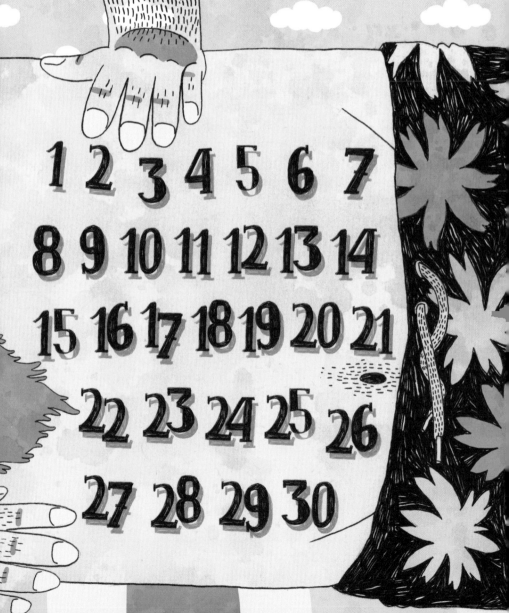

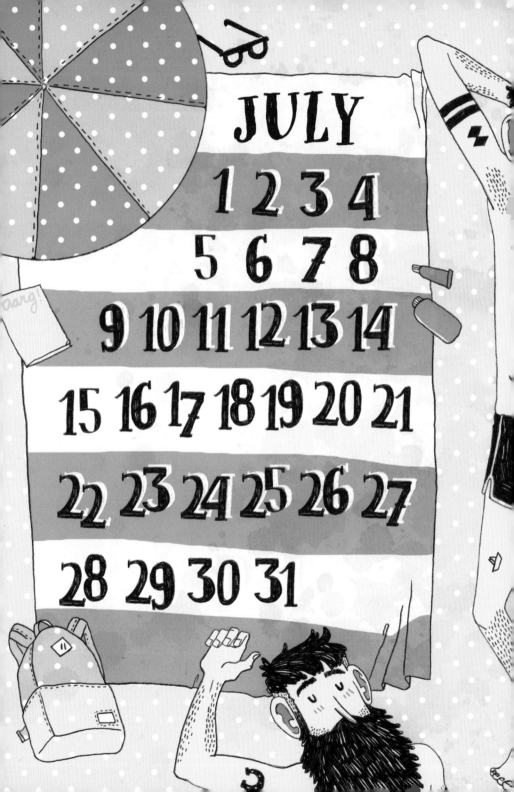

AUGUST

1 2 3 4 5 6 7
8 9 10 11 12 13 14
15 16 17 18 19 20 21
22 23 24 25 26 27
28 29 30 31

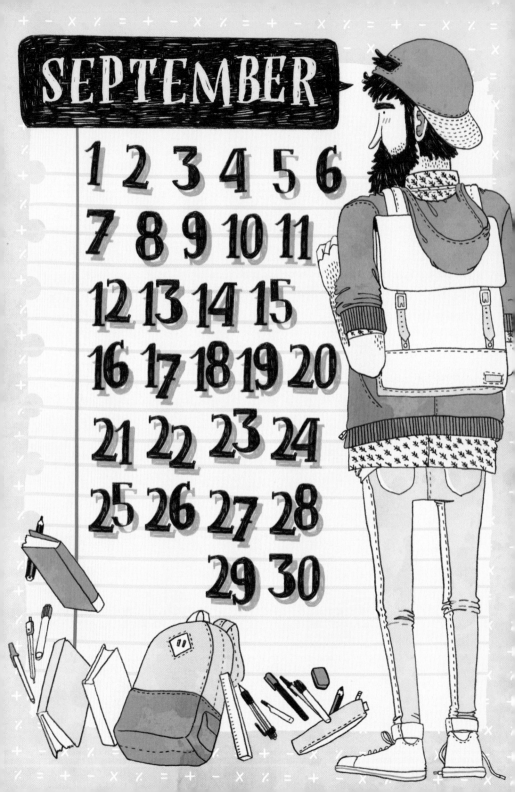

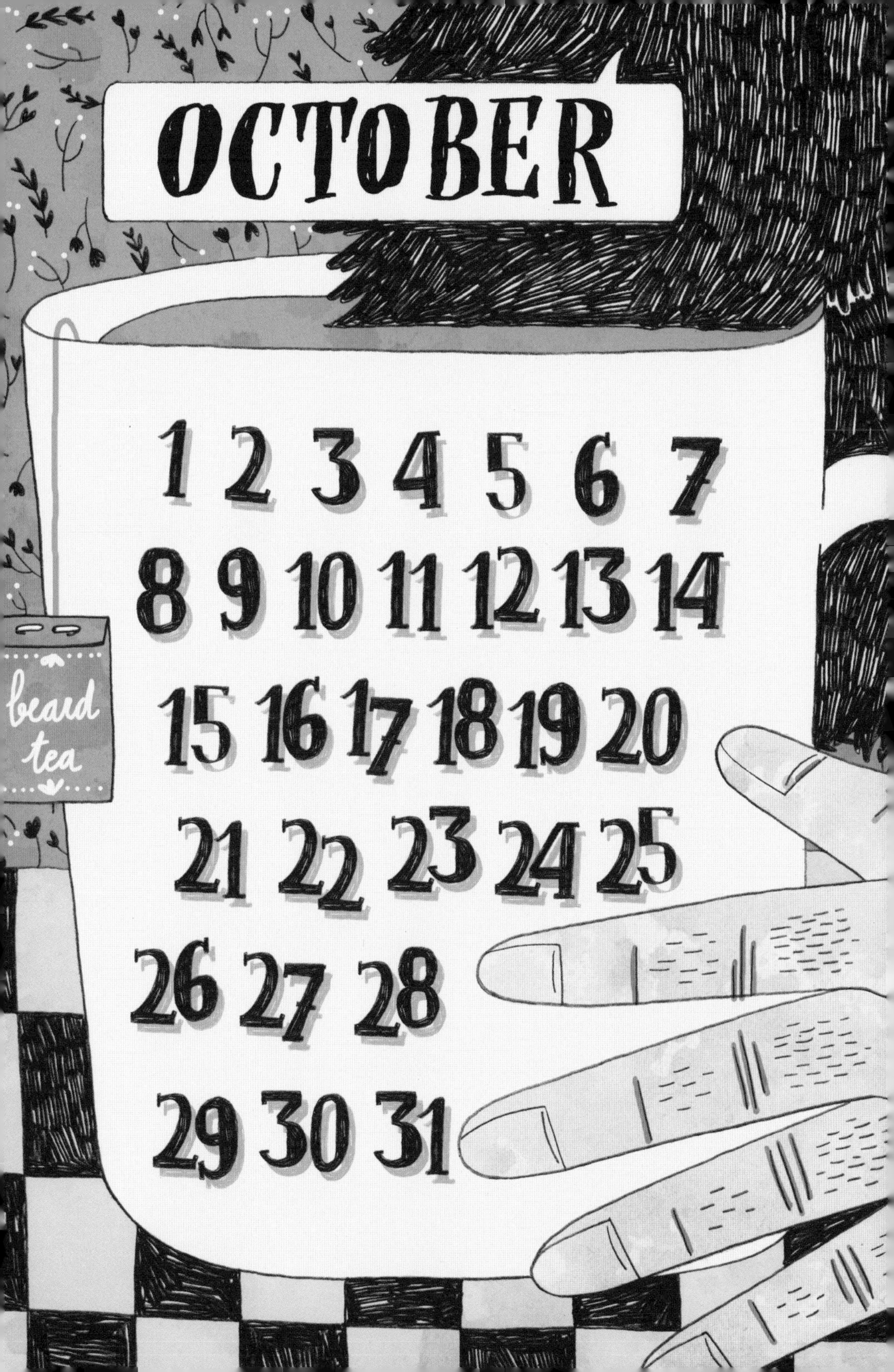
OCTOBER
1 2 3 4 5 6 7
8 9 10 11 12 13 14
15 16 17 18 19 20
21 22 23 24 25
26 27 28
29 30 31
beard tea

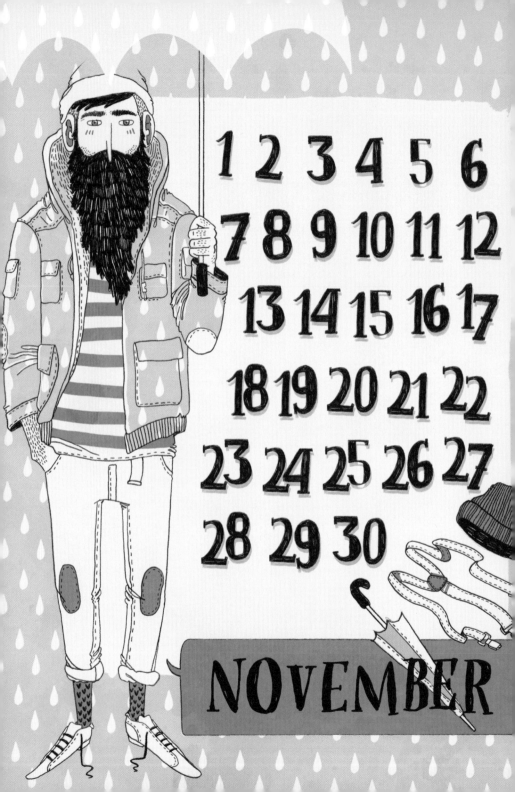

1 2 3 4 5 6
7 8 9 10 11 12
13 14 15 16 17
18 19 20 21 22
23 24 25 26 27
28 29 30

NOVEMBER

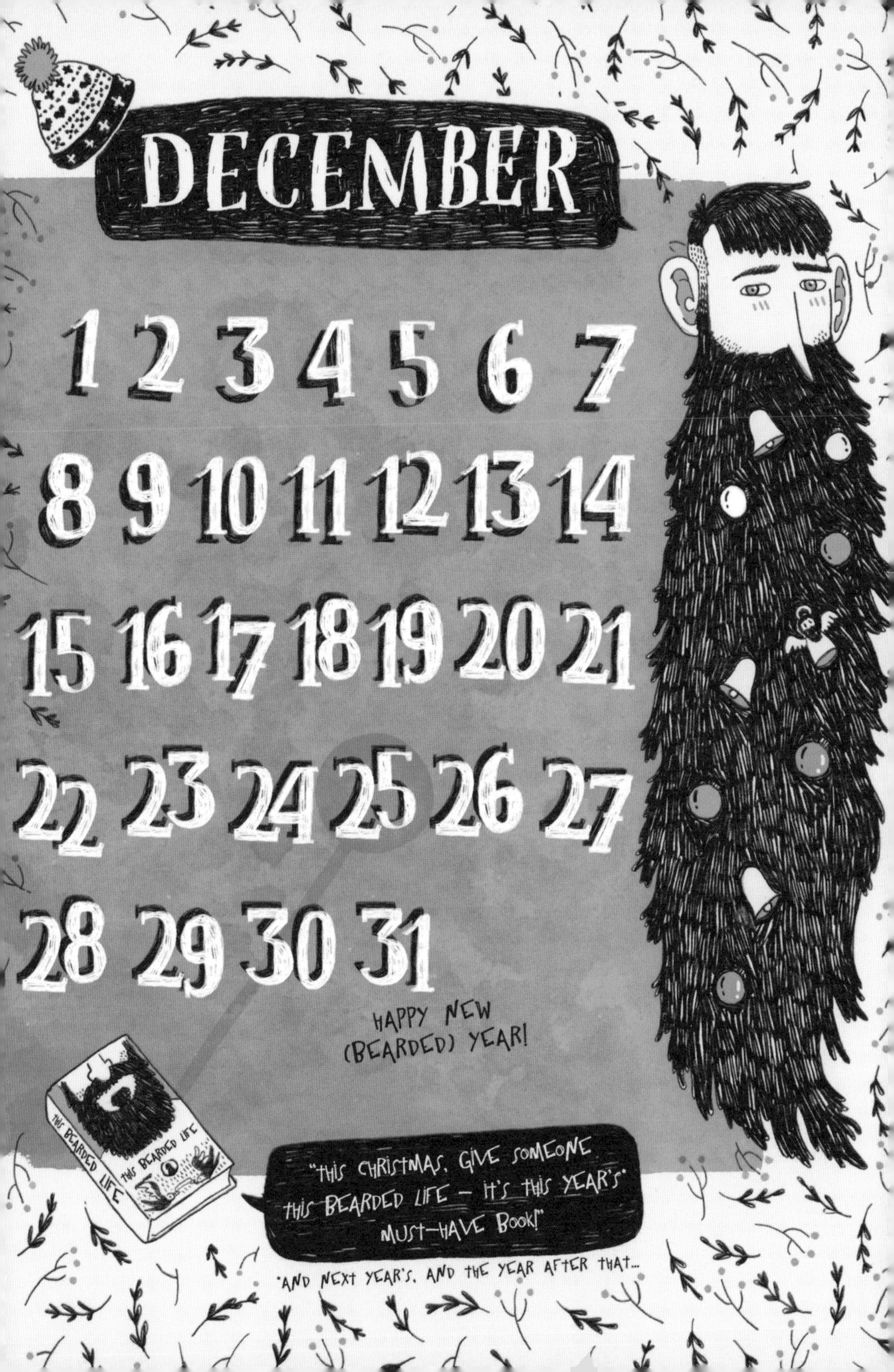

DECEMBER
1 2 3 4 5 6 7
8 9 10 11 12 13 14
15 16 17 18 19 20 21
22 23 24 25 26 27
28 29 30 31
HAPPY NEW (BEARDED) YEAR!
THIS BEARDED LIFE
THIS BEARDED LIFE
"THIS CHRISTMAS, GIVE SOMEONE THIS BEARDED LIFE – IT'S THIS YEAR'S* MUST-HAVE BOOK!"
*AND NEXT YEAR'S, AND THE YEAR AFTER THAT...

PHOTOGRAPHIC CREDITS

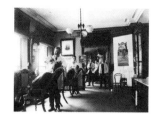

©IBL Bildbyra/Heritage Images/
Getty Images

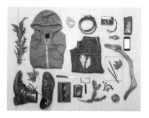

©Bonninstudio/Shutterstock.com

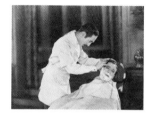

©Everett Collection/Shutterstock.com

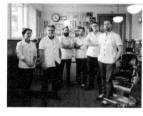

©New York Barbershop (Róterdam)

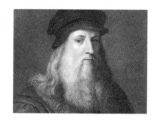

©Georgios Kollidas/Shutterstock.com

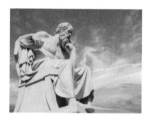

©Anastasios71/Shutterstock.com

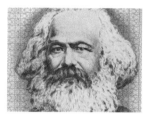

© Georgios Kollidas/Shutterstock.com

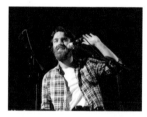

©Future-Image/Zumapress.com/
Album

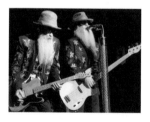

©TDC Photography/Shutterstock.com

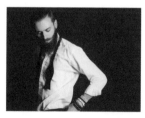

©Arthur Hidden/Shutterstock.com

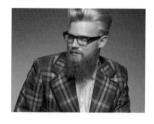

© Viorel Sima/Shutterstock.com

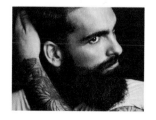

©Sfio Cracho/Shutterstock.com

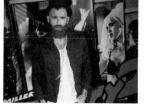

© 2014 Rex Features

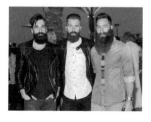

©Stefanie Keenan/Getty Images

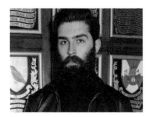

©David M. Benett/Getty Images

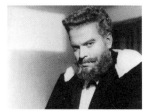

©Mercury/Cervantes Films/ Filmorsa/Album

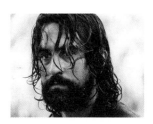

©Mondadori Portfolio/Album

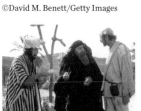

© Monty Python Films / The Kobal Collection

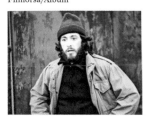

©Paramount Pictures/Album

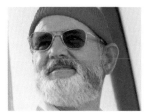

©Touchstone Pictures/Album

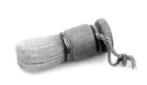

©Mondadori Portfolio/Album

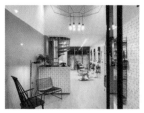

©Barbershop (Logroño)

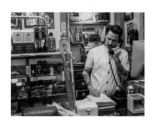

©Sabine Braun/Laif/Cordon Press

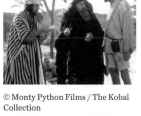

©Peter Zijlstra/Shutterstock.com

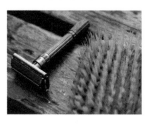

©Kevin Russ/Getty Images

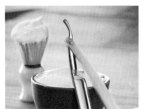

©Stuart Murray/Getty Images

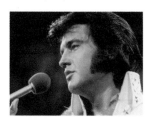

©Gary Null/NBC/NBCU Photo Bank/ Getty Images

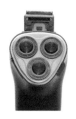

©Sergey Ash/Shutterstock.com

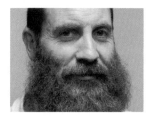

©Beautifulday/Shutterstock.com

ACKNOWLEDGEMENTS

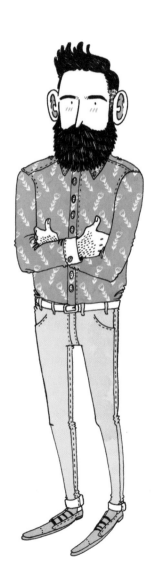

'TO CHARBEL, TO THE ALBERTOS, TO DARDO, MIREIA, ANDREA, SELIM, AND TO ALL THOSE I'VE FORGOTTEN: THIS BOOK IS YOURS TOO. THANK YOU ALSO TO LUNWERG FOR BELIEVING IN THIS HAIRY BOOK, AND TO ALFONSO FOR HIS ARTISTIC TALENT.

AND THANK YOU TO JORDI, FOR HIS ENDLESS PATIENCE!'

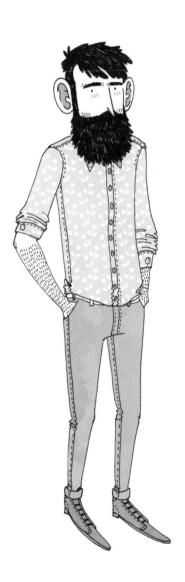

'TO JAVIER AND MIREIA, FOR OPENING THE DOORS OF THEIR HOUSE TO ME AND LETTING IT BECOME MY OWN.

TO CARLES, FOR RELYING ON ME AND FOR ALWAYS TREATING ME SO VERY WELL.

TO JORDI, FOR PUTTING UP WITH MY 'LAYOUT SUGGESTIONS', AND FOR HELPING TO PRODUCE A BOOK THAT IS AS MUCH HIS AS OURS.

TO MY MOTHER, WHO, DESPITE NOT BEING THIS BOOK'S INTENDED AUDIENCE, WILL DOUBTLESS READ IT, AND WHO SAID TO ME MANY YEARS AGO, 'DON'T SHAVE YOUR BEARD OFF, ALFONSO – ANYTHING THAT COVERS YOUR FACE IS AN IMPROVEMENT.'

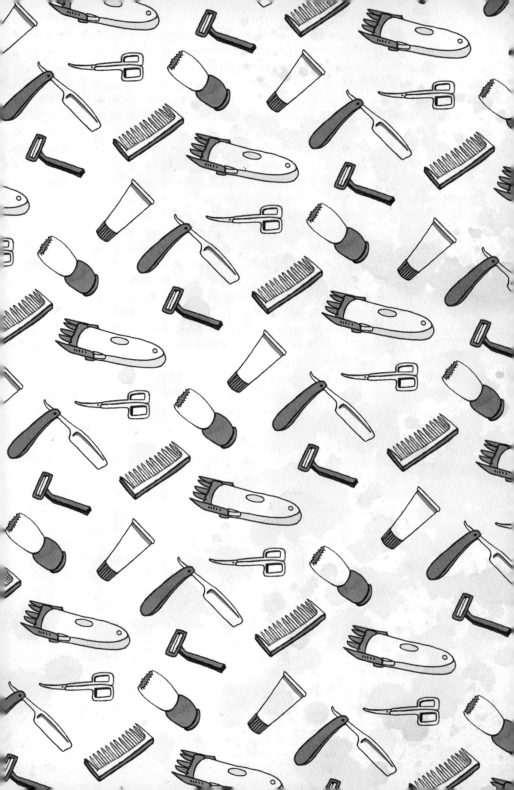